RAISING TEENS WITH DIABETES

A survival guide for parents

Moira McCarthy

with technical review by Jake Kushner, MD,
and Barbara J. Anderson, PhD

SpryPublishing
ideas to life

This edition is published by Spry Publishing LLC
2500 South State Street
Ann Arbor, MI 48104 USA

Printed and bound in the United States of America.

10 9 8 7 6 5 4 3 2 1

Library of Congress Control Number: 2013932653
Paperback ISBN: 978-1-938170-20-1
E-book ISBN: 978-1-938170-21-8

Who else but for Sean, Leigh, and Lauren,
who have been willing to take this crazy ride with me.
And to every "Diabetes Parent" out there.
We are family.

Contents

August 1989 was hot in Washington, D.C., really hot. Desperately hot. I remember Marissa, not quite two, playing on the swing set in the heat. She was thirsty—that was the heat, right? But she was thirsty at night, really thirsty, begging for water, all night and every night, for far too long. That wasn't the heat. That was something else. Just days after turning two, Marissa was diagnosed with type 1 diabetes.

My wife, Brenda, took Marissa to Children's National Medical Center, while I scrambled to return from a business trip. At Children's, we were lucky—very lucky—to be seen by a pediatric diabetes team, who told us, basically, not to worry and that everything would be OK. We had a great diagnosis experience, one that would guide us as Marissa grew up and that put our family on a path to share our experiences, many years later, through Children with Diabetes.

Today, nearly 24 years later, Marissa is grown-up. She graduated with a Bachelor's of Science in Nursing, passed the state boards to earn an RN, and married Adam, whom she met in nursing school. Marissa and Adam live close to Brenda and me; they work at a beautiful new hospital just down the road; and we spend a fair amount of time together as a family. And our daughter is perfectly healthy. For what more could we possibly ask?

As parents, we have one important job—helping our children grow up to become happy, healthy adults. Type 1 diabetes makes that job more challenging. What should be simple is not. For younger kids, you worry about care at school (who will be there if something happens?), how to take care of sleepovers, helping young friends understand diabetes, helping grandparents overcome their fears, among many things. For teens, you worry about care at school (will they remember to check blood sugars and take their insulin?), driving, peer pressure, dating, and what in the world to do about college. Add in the normal tension that comes from adolescence and you have the makings of potentially serious issues.

That's where Moira McCarthy's Raising Teens with Diabetes *comes in. Moira opens her heart to us, sharing her family's experiences helping her daughter Lauren through her teenage years. With kind, knowing wisdom and a wry wit, Moira takes on the task of helping us to navigate adolescence with type 1 diabetes. Whether your teen was recently diagnosed or your family has been living with type 1 diabetes for years, you'll find much to learn here. Confused about the various insulins available? Moira will help you consider the options. Injection therapy or an insulin pump? Check—and why not both? Continuous sensors? Yep. What about the impact of diabetes on family dynamics? Well cov-*

ered. Consider Raising Teens with Diabetes *as your compass and Moira as your captain through the potentially rough seas of the teenage years with type 1 diabetes.*

The suggestions and strategies within these pages will yield the best results if they are shared with your spouse, partner, and other adults with whom you share the responsibility of shepherding your teen to adulthood. It's not so much presenting a united front. It's more that these suggestions and strategies are valuable and can help enormously, so it's important for everyone to understand them and use them—and that includes your teen. There's no reason not to share and discuss Moira's wisdom with your teen. Chances are, they want to do well with their diabetes care, just like you want them to.

In my many years of leading Children with Diabetes, I have had the great fortune to meet some amazing people. Two are worth noting—Will Cross and Sebastien Sasseville, both of whom have type 1 diabetes. These two gentlemen have climbed to the top of Mt. Everest. I dare say that if you can climb to the top of the world with type 1 diabetes, there truly are no limits to what you can do.

JEFF HITCHCOCK
Founder and President, Children with Diabetes

When my daughter with diabetes was about eleven, I knew I had it all figured out. In fact, if I could have chosen a moniker, it absolutely would have been "Master of T1D!" (with a seldom-used-by-me exclamation point because, gosh darn it, I was the Master!). My daughter was the model patient. She checked when I needed her to. She bolused like a champ. She did all her own site changes and shots and all that kind of stuff. I was her "personal assistant," logging blood glucose values, studying charts to make changes in doses, keeping the insurance cads at bay. Clearly, she'd been listening to me since her diagnosis at six years old. Yep, we had it all down.

I felt sorry for some of my friends with older kids with type 1 diabetes (T1D). They struggled. Their kids rebelled. Their A1Cs skyrocketed. "I'm so glad," I thought to myself (with more than a moderate dose of "I'm just a great Mom" smugness), "that I raised Lauren not to be like that."

What I should have been thinking is this: Be careful what you crow about. Because in a heartbeat, it all can change.

That's what happened when the teen years hit. Seemingly out of the blue, Lauren's life with diabetes changed. Part of it was hormones: her body was playing games with her that even a crackerjack medical team could not figure out. Part of *it was my own burnout: when she moved toward indepen-dence with her disease it was easy for me to think "she's got this," when in fact she was not ready. Another part of it was free will: her brain was playing games with her diabetes that shook me to the core and, since I had little clue it was happening, sent her on a downward spiral that bottomed out in an intensive care unit.*

There she lay, tubes in arms, trying with all her heart to tell her mother and her doctors that she'd done this to herself. But each time she opened her mouth, someone else popped in to remark about the "model patient" and how her pump must have broken, or insulin must have gone bad, or the like. She told me later she didn't have the heart to steer us all right. She didn't want to let us down. Eventually, the labs told the story and she fessed up. She'd somehow lost her way with diabetes. She'd been lying and faking and skipping boluses and more. Once she told me, the clues were all lined up in front of me. I should have known. I should have seen. But I didn't.

I vowed to never let her land in the ICU again. I was successful with that (although not without many close calls). I vowed, too, to find all the resources I could on teens and diabetes, to read, read, read, and learn how to help her through this time.

And here's what I found: just about nothing. There was a

sea of info on raising children with T1D. There were quite a few books for adults. Our pediatric group seemed well equipped for kid stuff (and we loved them), but not as on top of the teen issues. I felt alone. And so I did my best to figure this all out as we went along, talking to other parents of teens with T1D, comparing notes, working on what helped and what did not.

Eventually, we came through. My daughter is now a vibrant, successful young adult who might even be a "model patient," if one takes into account what that means for a young adult. We survived the teen years, with all the horrifying twists and turns, all the crazy-town scares and freak-outs, and all the moments when it all seemed just impossible. I learned, slowly, how to not let my own fears rob her of her freedom. And she learned, slowly, how to not let her freedom put her in a place that we'd fear.

And now, it's my time to share all that. I am no Harvard-educated endocrinologic expert. In fact, rather than PhD after my name, I have a simple MOM. But it counts for something. And since I have an amazing team of medical experts backing my every word here, I feel confident that I can help.

Because, in all our years of T1D and teen-hood, I learned this: I am no superhero. Nor did I need to be. By sticking beside my daughter for better and worse; by adapting as she went along instead of stubbornly sticking to what worked when she was a preteen; by working on harnessing my own selfish fear of letting her spread her wings; by listening and learning, and then taking all that and reshaping it to my teen's needs, I helped her and me—and our entire family—not just survive but thrive.

So I'm hoping if you are a parent in need as I was back on that dark day, you've looked around, found this book, and now know that you are not alone. Because, no matter what the other parents may be saying about how their children are doing, you are not the only parent struggling with your teen.

Here's hoping that this book and the advice in it help you fare better, turn things sooner, and master life with diabetes with your teen sooner even than we did. There is power in information as well as in support. I hope you find both in these pages.

CHAPTER ONE

The Physiology of the Teen Years

I remember the moment we knew puberty was coming with our first child (my daughter without diabetes). I was away on business on the Alabama coast, playing a golf course to review it for a magazine. Hurricane Georges was bearing down on the very course I was playing on, and I was worrying about evacuation routes (while still playing as many holes as I could before they pulled us off). Back home in Massachusetts, my husband was watching the kids and facing down another impending storm: Hurricane Hormone. We'd both noticed how our quiet, compliant first child had become more, well, moody would be a polite word for it. And as I drove tees that morning, he noticed something else and called me about it.

"I had to take Leigh out and buy her some deodorant today!" he said almost breathless. Being the kind of wife I am, I saw this as a perfect "Punk!" opportunity and responded in a voice that feigned sincerity and concern. "Oh my goodness, Sean. Do you know that they usually get their first period within 24 hours of needing deodorant?" Mean prankster me could hear his brain cells crackling on the other end of the line. He paused a moment and then said this: "Get. Home. NOW. Holy Sh##!"

Of course I told him I was joking, and, of course, she did not get her period that very day. But wouldn't it be nice if puberty were that easy to detect, pinpoint, understand, and prepare for? It's not. With all children, we look for signs. In girls, it's the "puffy look" they get when they are changing from sprouting child to burgeoning young lady. In boys, it's cracks in the voice and hairs popping out here and there. But none of it is an exact science.

Throw diabetes into the mix, and you've really got a lot to grapple with. Are elevated blood sugars hints of hormone surges, or just the result of a few extra taco chips in the bowl? Is that grumpy attitude the result of hormones playing games with their mood, or are they going low? Or could it be a combination of both?

One thing is for sure: While diabetes makes it all more complicated and intense, for the most part, puberty does present itself in pretty much the same ways in kids with and without diabetes. We were lucky in that we had one daughter go through it without diabetes first. We were able to recognize what might be diabetes related and what was just plain "Hurricane Hormone." This chapter walks you through the basics of what to look for and what to expect.

And by the way, Alabama is a great place to play golf. But not during a hurricane warning.

The times (and the body and the mind and the psyche), they are a changin'. Okay, that's not quite how the old folk ballad went, but it could very well be the ballad for puberty. The puberty years are challenging for parents and children of all types. But with diabetes along for the ride, that ride can be even rougher.

First things first: Parents need to realize off the bat that millions and millions of adults are people with T1D who have lived through the adolescent years with diabetes onboard. True, it's more stressful and can even be scary at times, but diabetes and puberty are completely survivable. Most teens with diabetes come through unscathed and without complications, even if their road was a remarkably rough one. Parents fare worse: the worries and anguish may very well be the leading cause of gray hair (or so it feels). Knowing puberty is beginning, understanding the signs, and having a grasp on how to delve into all this is a great tool, one that can help a parent—and a teen—better navigate these choppy waters.

Puberty in General—Signs and Average Ages

Puberty is a sneaky little thing. If only we could pinpoint its arrival the same way we can the start of school years. But we cannot. And like so many other things in parenting, the arrival of true puberty is unique to each and every child.

That said, medical experts can point to a period of time in your children's lives when they are most likely to start puberty. For girls, the average age for puberty to commence runs from ages 9 to 13. For boys, most medical experts say things start up between ages 9 and 14.

For girls, the first noticeable signs come once something we cannot see—estrogen—begins pumping through their bodies. Once estrogen begins pumping, girls usually show signs such as the beginning of breast buds, increase in hair on arms and legs, appearance of hair under arms and in private areas, and a noticeable increase in speed for additional height and weight (that quick weight is what many parents notice as a "puffy period," when girls just look more puffy). Body odor is another sign. Once you've purchased that deodorant and shown your daughter how to use it because she really needs it, you can be sure that puberty has begun. Periods come later in puberty, with experts saying the average age for a first period is around 12 or 13. Some say this age is decreasing, but for now, medical experts point to that time as the average age.

For boys, the hormone that puts it all into play is testosterone. Once testosterone increases in a boy's body, boys experience increased growth in height, weight, and shoulder width. In fact, a "sprouting" in height and widening of shoulders is often the first sign parents have that boys are in puberty. Boys, too, will be able to use body odor as a pinpoint for puberty, and everyone knows that increased testosterone affects the larynx, leading to voice cracking and eventually deepening, which is probably the best-known aspect of puberty for boys. Boys develop more hair as well on their arms, legs, chest, armpits, private areas, and, of course, face.

So what does all that mean with diabetes onboard? All kinds

of variables. It can be a challenge for parents to figure out when it's the hormones, when it's the diabetes, and when it's both.

Some things are known. According to medical experts, teens have a 1 percent higher average blood glucose (BG) compared with adults, which means they typically require more insulin. As noted, the key to puberty are those sex hormones. Those hormones in all of us work against insulin, rather than with it. While insulin lowers blood sugars, sex hormones work to elevate blood sugars. If this sounds like a battle going on inside your teen's body, that's about right. The body in puberty sees a decrease in insulin activity by as much as 30 to 50 percent, which contributes to higher glucose levels and an increased need for insulin. And that's just the physical aspect. When you consider this is an age when children with diabetes crave freedom and self-sufficiency, and just plain want to be kids, it's easy to see why challenges abound for both parents and teens.

Is the Average Age of Puberty Decreasing?

According to the respected journal *Pediatrics*, more and more American and European girls, particularly Caucasians, are showing signs of breast buds and the start of puberty at a younger age, sometimes as young as seven. The reason is still being studied. Some hint it may be hormones in food, while others point to higher obesity rates. The average age, though, still stands at what is mentioned here.

For Girls—What It All Means Diabetes-Wise

Diabetes overlaps with everything our teens do in life and, in puberty, that can be extra challenging for girls. First, there is, of course, The Big M: menstrual cycles. Managing diabetes during a menstrual cycle is a whole new variable for teens with diabetes and their caretakers. Some girls experience spikes in glucose levels, requiring additional insulin during this time. Other girls find the strain on the body actually leads to a decrease in the need for insulin, much in the same way exercise or exertion can. Only time and experience help girls find out how this impacts them.

Why? Insulin works by attaching or "binding to" protein receptors on the surface of cells. Once it binds, that allows the cells to use glucose for fuel (the insulin is like the gate key for the glucose to get in). Some studies show that when progestin hormones are high, as they can be before and during a menstrual cycle, this process can be compromised somewhat, leading to insulin resistance and, therefore, higher blood sugars.

Some teens also experience bloating, water retention, and, of course, food cravings during this time (particularly carbs!), which can lead to elevated blood sugars as well. But some females experience no impact at all on their blood sugars during this time of the month. How will you know where your daughter falls in that wide spectrum?

The best thing a parent and teen can do is gather information. From the time menstrual cycles begin, try to do a few extra blood glucose checks each day and log them for study and comparison. And here's a tip: do *not* make changes based on what you see in one cycle. Rather, gather information from at least three (or even more) cycles and look for patterns, then make changes. This may be a good time to ask your certified diabetes educator (CDE) or endocrinologist to weigh in as well.

Of course, the irony here is that with most girls (with diabetes or not) the *last* thing they want to do is call attention to their periods, much less study them up

A Tried and True Book Still Works

It's nearly 50 years old, but the fact of the matter is that *Are You There, God? It's Me, Margaret* still works as an excellent discussion tool and educational piece for girls waiting on their first period. Buy it, reread it, and then have your daughter read it. Judith Blume still works so well.

close. And girls with diabetes tend to want *less* diabetes details in the teen years, not more. Parents should begin explaining to their preteen girl at as young an age as possible that all this will be worked out. While the first periods may take some extra attention, in time you'll know what goes on (for the most part) and know how to deal with them blood sugar–wise. Try to let her know that, unlike some other parts of her life with diabetes, this will not be shared, that you understand her need for privacy, and you will respect that as you work through this time with her.

So what do you do with that information? Ask your medical team for help and look for hints to determine if you need to cut back or add on to the basal insulin (basal rate if on a pump; long acting if on injections). In most cases, the changes will come in the basal and long acting, since the period occurs over time and is not a short event like a meal. It will be a good idea to keep a calendar for periods and related information for a year or so, separate from any you have for life or diabetes in general. The sooner you can help your daughter understand that she can take some action if periods throw her diabetes off, the sooner you are helping her see she does not have to be a victim to them. In some cases, changes may not be made at all. If you and your team find the spikes and swings are too unpredictable during that time of the month, you may decide to just change your goals for that time. It's something to think about and discuss as a team, with your daughter at the center of that team.

One of the most important things to remember from the start is simple: don't scare your daughter about it. Instead of saying that a period could cause crazy blood sugar swings (because they might not—each female is unique), tell her that it's a time you need to pay extra attention to so you can make sure she is happy and comfortable. But also be sure she knows that if she does experience highs or lows she does not understand during those days of the month, she should not beat herself up about them. Rather, she should discuss them with you so you can figure out a plan. And sometimes, highs are just going to happen. Be sure your daughter knows that so long as you work at correcting them, highs are not going to hurt her. You, as a parent, need to embrace this, too. While we work—every day—to avoid highs, sometimes (like during a period) they happen in spite of our greatest effort. Correct and move on. That's your best bet.

Weight gain is another issue with which teen girls can grapple. With the social pressure to be thin assaulting girls from almost every angle, with popular clothing stores stocking tighter and tighter fits, and with pop culture celebrating the emaciated, girls are bound to be racked with body image issues at this age. Without diabetes onboard, estrogen causes some weight gain. In addition, as the body changes and develops, most healthy girls develop curves. This can be stressful for any adolescent girl.

Once again, diabetes adds to the dilemma. (More details on this and on dangerous eating issues can be found in chapter 13.) Because here's the rub: with an increased need for insulin spurred by the estrogen pulsing through their bodies, girls with diabetes are also experiencing the weight gain that comes with puberty. This is like a double whammy, and the concept that this may be a temporary thing falls on deaf ears. That is why this time is ripe for girls (and boys, for that matter) to develop eating disorders.

> **Clothing Sizes Can Hurt**
>
> Be sure to show your daughter or son that clothing sizes differ from store to store and that what matters is how something feels on you. Consider cutting the size tags out of their clothes when they purchase them. That way they won't fret if they think they're in a size they "should not be in."

What is a parent to do? The good news about this age is that it is the time girls—and boys—are considering what sports teams they want to join. If your child is an athlete, encourage him or her to step up the training for a sport. For non-athletes, encourage them to try an activity. Exercise is the best option to fight the weight gain that comes with puberty. Exercise also helps the body better use insulin, which could mean a cutback in dosing and then less possibility of weight gain from insulin use. It's a good idea to try to encourage a teen with diabetes to live a life with exercise in it anyway. Here you have a chance to do it without attaching it to diabetes. Sports are part of many teen lives. Now is a great time to get your teen interested in one. And it can help.

You may want to ask your daughter's medical team to adjust their "goals" for her weight and height, too. The "normal" charts used to track growth can upset a teen girl with diabetes. Better yet, consider having the team not fill out that chart in front of your daughter. There is little need for her to know what percentile she is in. And remind your daughter: girls lie about their weight. All the time. Encourage her not to share hers and not to take it too seriously when other girls share theirs.

For Boys—What It All Means Diabetes-Wise

Some parents like to say boys with diabetes are easier to manage than girls with diabetes. Those who say that would be the parents of girls. True, boys don't have to deal with the "Big M," but they do have their own unique challenges as puberty comes along.

Testosterone is a powerful hormone, and many teen boys with T1D experience some shocking (to them and their parents) blood sugar swings. It can be confusing, frustrating, and even frightening when they swing from high to low and back again, all in a day's time. The best tool parents have is information. Since teen boys are working toward more freedom (and like to slam their bedroom doors shut and be alone much of the time), it can be a challenge for parents to stay on top of what is going on and make smart dosing decisions. Boys (and girls, too) will want to push their parents away at this time, saying they don't need help and can handle it alone. And while they probably can intellectually and possibly emotionally, too, it's best not to leave them to their own devices. This is the time in their lives, ironically, when they need you to intervene the most. While it may not be the best idea for you to be actually doing the checks, you should be part of them. Temptation is a powerful drug, and teens face it every single day. Whether it's to scarf down some corn chips and not bolus, or to just skip a dose here and there, or to "rage bolus" away a high, teens are tempted. Parents need to find a way to stay on top of what their sons (and daughters) are doing behind closed doors.

Boys, too, struggle with body image at this time and may find they are gaining weight in ways they just don't want to. Educate your son about hormones and insulin and why it might mean he could gain a few extra pounds for a little bit of time. And encourage him to delve into sports, too. Not only would getting a good run for the cross country team help his weight, it also can help his mood, as exercise is a natural mood enhancer.

This is the age, too, when boys start to think about sex. Thanks to the blight of TV advertisements for medication for erectile dysfunction (ED) (often during the football games and sports events boys love to watch), teen boys with and without diabetes are constantly exposed to the notion that someday their penis may not work.

Parents need to make sure their son knows early and knows

that he will most likely *not* suffer that complication. It sounds silly, but it weighs on the mind of teen boys. Explain to them that those commercials are for older men, many of whom don't even have T1D. Many of them grew up in a time when there were no meters, few choices of insulin, and a whole different standard of care than is available for your son today. He might flinch when you have the conversation, but have it. It's important he knows that ED is not a sure thing in his future and that, in fact, he'll most likely never deal with it.

Better a Son or Daughter with Diabetes? *Tom Karlya*

Having a son and a daughter with diabetes, and also having been part of the diabetes community for as long as I have, has allowed me to make certain personal observations. I did not want a "new normal" and still hate that it has taken up residence in our household. But it's here and we deal with it every day.

Many people have asked me if there is a difference between a daughter and a son having diabetes. Now, in reality, I believe what they are asking me, or what they are hoping for, is for me to grant some conventional wisdom as to whether it is better or worse if a male gets diabetes or if a female does. I know they really want to know if they are in for a road of hell or a road of exponentially worse hell.

If it will make anyone feel better, I do not think it really matters, and what I have witnessed may be completely different from what you will. I'm continually amazed at the resilience of kids in adapting: they truly are better than we are at moving forward. Where we think that our world, their world, and everything will fall apart now that diabetes has entered our lives, quite frankly, they just want to get back outside and play.

Take note: they just want to get back outside and play.

Keep your focus on that point. As much as you make a big deal about your child's diabetes, so will your child. If you make diabetes the center and most important and only thing in your life, so will your children. Get them "back outside to play" as fast as possible. Make that the rule in every area.

In teenage years, both girls and boys will try to just manage quickly. Checking blood sugars and adjusting pumps "and getting it done." Boys seem to be less conscious of wearing devices like pumps and continuous glucose monitors (CGMs) than girls, especially in the teen years. Boys will also be very creative in trying to hide worn diabetes devices in their sports equipment when needed. Don't get me wrong, they both *know* a device is there and are *very* aware it is attached to their body, but boys seem to deal with this aspect a bit better. This is an interesting contradiction, for boys are sometimes more likely to want to go to the boys' room and check blood sugars in a stall, whereas girls will just take out the glucometer and check their blood sugar, and continue on.

Of course, physically, young women have much more to deal with as they deal with hormonal changes once a month in addition to balancing highs and lows. This is particularly challenging, for it is also common for young women not to talk about anything, which leaves it up to us to guess what exactly a particular response is responding to. If it makes you feel any better, this time is not easy in any household, diabetes or not.

Whatever the age, in all cases continually remind yourself (if you do not have diabetes), you really do not know what it is like to have it. We don't. At any age, diabetes management is not like telling your kids to clean their room; if you treat it like that, your results will be the same as well.

It sounds like rhetoric to hear how important communication is when dealing with both boys and girls and their diabetes. I must share that we have found this to be very true. I have found that parents who have dealt with their kids' diabetes in an atmosphere of "working it out," and not making kids just do what they are told, usually fare better. Seek out a balance, and it will come.

Tom Karlya has two children with T1D and is known in the diabetes community as Diabetes Dad, his pen name for his blog (www.diabetesdad.org) and his articles (www.dlife.com/diabetesdad). He lectures globally, has testified in legislative sessions, has chaired panels, and writes to inspire others to "Not Do Nothing." He is presently the vice president of the Diabetes Research Institute Foundation (www.diabetesresearch.org) and resides on Long Island, New York. He can be contacted at tkarlya@drif.org.

Growth Spurts in Boys and Girls

One of the things parents anticipate—and dread—most in these years are growth spurts. For both boys and girls, growth hormones don't work on a straight line or even a bell curve. Rather, they spike, and dip, and spike again, with no clear rhyme or reason. And since growth hormones can affect how insulin (also a hormone) works in the body, it can be challenging for parents.

When growth hormones are surging through your child's body, he or she may develop a temporary need for increased insulin, not just in long-acting, but in rapid-acting as well. The problem is figuring out how much and when. Since diabetes is all about looking for patterns and then making adjustments, this is a time when that can be a challenge. Talk to your endocrinology (endo) team about it and see if they want you to react to growth spurts with increased insulin. (A rare few teens react to growth spurts with lows, so a decrease might even be a possibility.)

The first thing you need to do is make sure the high (or low) is actually caused by the growth hormones. Remember, this is a time when your teen is grazing food more, eating out with friends, forgetting to bolus sometimes, and guessing on carbs. It's a real irony that the time you need to truly know what is going on in the body is also the time when your child may not always be under your wing or keeping an eye on the diabetes ball.

Once you are relatively sure that growth hormones may be the culprit, talk to your team. But don't be surprised if their answer is to just let it be. Drastic changes in an insulin plan are usually not made on random happenings. And unfortunately, growth spurts are random. It's frustrating, to be sure, but your team should encourage you that this is a short time and that it, too, will pass. And, sometimes, since the spikes from this are truly out of your teen's control, trying too hard to avoid them may lead to your teen feeling like a failure—something you do not want to happen.

The Start of Mood Swings (And How to Deal with Them)

Admit it: in the past, you judged another parent when you saw a teenager pitching a hissy fit. You might have been in the market or with them at a family party. When you saw the teen talk in a mean tone, freak out about something silly, or just plain be rude, you said to yourself (as you looked at your polite, sweet, soft-spoken nine-year-old), "Well, I'm glad I didn't raise my child like that."

Because none of us, really, raise our kids to not act appropriately. We start from day one teaching them to be kind, polite, calm, and reasonable. But what we don't know is what we learn quickly as puberty commences: mood swings are hard to avoid.

It can be shocking the first time parents see it in a child, when their sweet little girl suddenly goes all Linda Blair, or their son channels Damien. Because when it happens with your child, it's not fiction, and it's hard to joke about it.

It's important to accept, first, that some mood swings and erratic behavior are actually physical. People like to joke that teens have not fully formed their frontal lobes yet, but that's no joke. In fact, the last part of the brain that develops physically is the prefrontal cortex. This is the part of the brain responsible for self-control, judgment, and planning. So while we adults struggle with our moods at times, teens have a bit of a reason for being moody: their brains are still developing. So, in a way, when they shout, "It's not fair! It's not my fault!" they are partially right.

But still, teens have to learn to cope with all this onboard. After all, they cannot just go around raging and screaming and pitching fits. And learning to cope is possible. The anthropologist Margaret

Mood Swings and You: Modeling for Your Child

Even parents have mood swings and outbursts. Now is the time to learn to control yours or make the right apologies or adjustments after you have one. Show your child that you, too, are human and fall from grace from time to time. Seeing that and how you recover can help them learn to do the same. If you freak out, fess up. And make right.

Mead did extensive studies on teens in cultures around the globe and found that cultural, spiritual, and familial factors could play a role in mood swings (or the lack thereof). But can you remove them completely? Probably not. And Mead never, as far as we know, studied them in teens with diabetes, who also face blood sugar fluctuations that can mess with a mood as well.

The reality is that almost all teens experience mood swings and have a hard time controlling them. When you add diabetes to the equation, parents end up wondering: is it a high or low blood sugar, or just moods? Or a mix of both?

So here is the solution: it does not matter. As teens begin to get sullen and moody, it is important for parents to teach them about controlling emotions, finding ways to work them out appropriately, and behaving well in public, as well as in private. Because the reality is: diabetes or no diabetes, your goal is to raise a person who can fare well in the "real world." Knowing how to handle mood swings is a part of that goal.

It's important to be calm when a teen rips into a mood swing. If it's a loud one, with shouting and arguing, you need to do all you can to *not* argue back or shout back (easier said than done). Your child is looking to stir things up and looking for a reaction in you to justify theirs. So, your first line of defense is simple: remain calm. Do not take the bait. Instead, remind your child of some coping methods you've discussed in advance. Some ideas include:

- Create a "calm-down space" for your teen to go to when

moody and upset. Some choose their bedrooms, others choose a comfortable chair in a room where they are alone. Agree that if your child lashes out and then heads to that place, you will let them be until they've calmed down enough to have a semi-rational discussion.

- Encourage your teen to use exercise to work out a mood. A walk, a run, even some time on the swing set (teens still like them) can give them some cool-down time when upset.
- Journaling. It sounds silly, but getting them to go sit down and write out their grievances can be healing. And it's their choice if you read it or not when they are done. Writing is a slower process than yelling. It helps teens stop and think about what they are upset about, and helps that unfinished part of the brain catch up to what is or is not going on.
- Encourage—and accept—apologies. Teens are often afraid to say they are sorry about an outburst. First of all, saying "sorry" is acknowledging that it happened in the first place. Like toddlers, teens want to use wishful thinking to make it all just go away. Second, sometimes a teen may have to apologize multiple times a day. No matter how upset you are or how many times you've heard "sorry" that day, accept it. That's a powerful lesson for life.

So what about blood sugars and moods? Parents ask all the time: should my teen be held accountable for an outburst or snarky comment he or she made when blood sugar was high or low? The answer, simply, is yes.

Okay, so it does not seem fair. Your teen did not ask for T1D and often cannot help being high or low. But here's the thing: your job as a parent is to raise your teen to be a useful, responsible, and agreeable adult in the outside world. The reality is, until there is a cure, your child needs to learn to do that with T1D onboard. There will be few—or no—free passes for their behavior in the world, and you have to help them learn what to do when a high or a low causes them to act out in a moody way. Besides the suggestions above, teens will need to remember that the best thing they can do if a high or a low sends them into a mood swing is *correct their blood sugar*. Of course, in that moment, this is the last thing they want to hear from you. Parents need to get teens to understand that if they feel that it might be a high (and usually highs cause more angst), then checking, correcting, and using the steps above is their best bet. And while diabetes may have been "to blame," apologies are still in order.

It's also hard for parents to remember this: a rational discussion with a moody teen in the middle of a high blood sugar is near impossible. So the best thing you can do as a parent is encourage them to quiet down, be alone, and turn things around.

The good news with all of this is that puberty passes, and so do many of the mood swings. One day your son or daughter will be an adult and, just as with childbirth, you'll forget all the moody moments and hard times and swear up and down that he or she was an absolutely agreeable teen.

That's because the brain is a mysterious, wonderful tool that does that for us, too. Thank goodness for our own semi-flawed frontal lobes.

CHAPTER TWO

Diabetes and the Newly Diagnosed Teen

What is the "best age" to be diagnosed with T1D? It's a question parents in the diabetes world ask one another all the time. Is it better to have been diagnosed as a young child ("they don't know any different way of life") or better as a teen ("they can understand it all and take on responsibility right away")? Here's my response: there is no good time to be diagnosed with T1D. Children who start a life with diabetes at a young age are often burned out in the teen years. They also have had the clock ticking on them longer. Even in this era of reduced diabetes complications, there are still things that just plain wear on the body. Shot or pump sites, for example. As the years go on, sites become used up, and less real estate is available to inject or place a pump.

Fingertips become callous and worn, a visual representation of the years with diabetes. Kids—and parents—just plain get sick of it.

And as for being newly diagnosed in the teen years, well, to me that just seems like a cruel trick. For children at that age it is more important to fit in and begin to gain freedom from parents, moving toward a more individual life. Along comes T1D and it can feel, to the teen, like none of that will ever happen. Adding to the situation is the fact that teens are not with their parents every moment, as they are as little kids, and that can make adapting to a new life with T1D all the more stressful.

A new diagnosis can send a family into a tailspin, no matter what the age. For my family, it was at a semi-young age. (Lauren had just started kindergarten when the diagnosis came. In hindsight, she could have been diagnosed a few weeks prior.) Today, she says she's glad she was younger, that she has a special place in her heart for the newly diagnosed teen. But I think that's just her being a good sport about it all. In the end, kids with T1D become adept at convincing themselves they are okay and others have it worse. They also seem to sprout extra strands of compassion. They get it. They feel it. They live it. And for that reason, they always think the other person has it harder.

If you are the parent of a newly diagnosed teen, I hope

this chapter helps you. And I hope your teen's diagnosis brings you closer together rather than driving you apart. I can tell you this: going through the teen diabetes years with my daughter was a crazy challenge, but a challenge that made our relationship all the stronger. It wasn't all happiness and joy, but it was all caring and moving toward teamwork. Here's wishing that for you.

A diabetes diagnosis always comes as a shock and often comes seemingly out of nowhere. And while the highest percentage of diagnoses of diabetes comes in the puberty years, parents can be taken quite by surprise. Why? First off, preteens and teens don't spend as much time with their parents. They leave early for school and often have after-school activities that keep them from home until close to dinnertime. Parents can't notice possible symptoms such as extra trips to the rest room or excessive thirst because their child is not with them all day long.

Second, it's easy as a parent to kind of "settle in" on the physical things about raising a child at this point. You've been through the baby and toddler years. You know what their educational needs are. You can see the light at the end of the tunnel: adulthood.

This is an age where the very basic symptoms of the onset of T1D can be confused with other things, too. A girl drops weight quickly. Could that be an eating disorder? A teen chugs down gallons of milk or juice each day. Could they be letting themselves dehydrate at sports practice? Exhaustion? With sports and school and stress and life in general, it's tiring being a teen these days. Even the vomiting that can come with extended high blood sugars can be blamed on something else.

But here's the thing: if you did see symptoms you blamed on

something else and now realize in hindsight were due to T1D, don't beat yourself up. As of now, there is nothing, *nothing*, you could have done to stop the onset of the disease. All you can do now is make sure children understand that anything going on in their bodies at that time—including bed-wetting, which teens sometimes hide from their parents out of embarrassment—was not their fault. And now you're ready to figure out just how they are going to live their lives richly and fully with T1D onboard.

"Like a New Baby"

Having a teen diagnosed with diabetes can feel like you felt the first time you brought a baby home—only this time you did not plan for it. Give yourself time to adjust, adapt, and understand, just like you did when you first brought your baby home.

Looping Parents in from the Start

When a child is small, it's important that parents are educated on every aspect of T1D when a child is diagnosed. After all, the parent/caretaker will be that child's lifeline once they leave the hospital. But with teens, that can be tricky. Some teens want to take control of the situation from the start. However, this should not be encouraged, given all the research that tells us that teens with T1D need their parents throughout adolescence, just in a different way. Parents need to make sure they are completely in the loop and understand everything there is to know about their teen's diabetes. Why? Because while teens may feel independent and up for it, they are going to need their parents as backup and support.

If your teen is newly diagnosed, here are some tips to consider:
- Even if your teen is doing the blood glucose readings and shots, learn how to do them as well. You can practice on an orange (and most hospitals have fake butts to use, too). You can practice on yourself with saline if you ask the

doctor. And do give at least a couple of shots to your teen, just so you know you can do it. (And your teen will know you can do it, too.)

- Read, read, read. You already have this book in your hand, so you've started. But read all you can. See the appendix of this book for both online and print suggestions. Don't think that because a book is about raising a younger child you won't learn from it. Information is power.

- Insist on sharing blood glucose logging duties for at least the first six months. Tell your teen you want to do it for learning purposes, and be sure to help look for patterns and needed changes (discussed in chapter 4). This will also ensure you know how to use all the tools your teen is using, so you can take over care as a way of supporting him or her when needed.

Sharing with Family and Friends: A Unique Dynamic

Teens, for the most part, are secretive. And they want to feel "normal." So sharing the news of their diagnosis could be tricky. But there is one thing you must help your teen realize from the start: the sooner people know and the more people who know, the less of a big deal the diagnosis will be. True, people will be shocked and worried, but once that passes, most will follow your lead if you let them know this is going to be a part of your teen's life, and life is going to go on almost as it was before, just with some added medical duties.

So whose job is it to share? When it

> **Once Out, Not a Big Deal**
>
> It's hard for teens to grasp this, but the fact is that the sooner they share that they have diabetes and what it means, the less of a big deal it will be to other people. Encourage them to test this theory out. It's true.

comes to family, it's fair enough that you let your teen know that you will be making the family aware of what is going on and how they can help. A great idea is appointing a family member who is a good communicator to keep everyone up to date via email from the start. You'll want to show your teen what you're sending so they know what you are saying. Be sure to explain to all family members and friends exactly what T1D is and how it is different from type 2. Give them a basic overview of what your teen will be doing and learning over the coming months. And suggest some reading for them as well. Encourage them to learn about T1D so they can understand exactly what is going on, rather than be confused or say things that don't make sense or might be hurtful to your teen.

Teen Perspective, Madison Bingaman, diagnosed with T1D at age 17

"I didn't care that I had to give myself shots, count carbohydrates, or worry about my blood sugar. My health wasn't my problem. My problem was that I was now going to be a problem. My family, friends, and anyone else who came into my life would now have to learn about diabetes—all because of me. I didn't want people to have to learn about diabetes or even worry about me. No matter how many times someone told me they *wanted* to learn about it, I didn't believe them. I felt like a burden and problem for everyone surrounding me. As time went on, I got used to telling people that I had diabetes. Most, not all, would ask questions and show interest. Little did they know, I was awfully flattered and more than appreciative for their simply asking a question. I always heard the typical, "I couldn't do it" response—I still get it! When I hear it now, it is just part of my life and something I do every day."

As for their friends, it is up to the teen to tell them. But tell them he or she must. Your teen may want to host a get-together with his or her closest friends to explain the basics. You can even make it fun: a dinner party at which the friends can all see that your teen can still eat most foods and live life a "normal" way.

Helping those friends to "get it" from the start will pave the way for how things go at school, at sports, and out and about in life as a teen.

What about school? It is imperative that the school knows about your teen's diagnosis. You'll need to set up a meeting with the school nurse either the day before your child returns to school or the morning he or she returns. (We discuss how to handle the school nurse situation in chapter 7.) Teachers will need to be notified as well, and you'll need to discuss with your teen what their rights are in school with T1D onboard. Some teens balk at this, saying they'd rather fly under the radar and keep it to themselves. But again, it is imperative that everyone know your teen now has T1D. Have the medical team back up your stance that the more people know, the less of a big deal it is.

What about the teen who starts out wanting to be completely private about the diagnosis and who fights any discussion? It is your job as a parent to keep a teen safe, and you need to explain to your teen that part of keeping him or her safe is letting the school and good friends know what is going on. However, let teens know you will respect their privacy in any way that you can safely. If they don't want you blasting blood sugars or health updates on social media, respect that. If they don't want you telling strangers in the store, respect that, too.

Choosing a Method of Daily Care

Right off the bat, you and your teen will be working with the medical team to choose a method of care that might be confusing to you. In almost every case, a newly diagnosed person begins on multiple daily injections (MDIs). There is a discussion of different insulins and choices in chapter 4, but at the start, your team will probably suggest either a combination of NPH insulin and a rapid-acting insulin, or a combination of a longer-acting insulin such as Lantus and a rapid-acting insulin. The decision comes down to deciding if you want a treatment plan that is more similar to the working human pancreas or less similar. Here is what you need to know: there are many, many choices in methods of care now, and you can make changes at any time.

It is important that teens feel they can make this decision with their medical team. While parents—and the medical team most of all—should absolutely have input, the teen is the one who must "own" (and therefore accept) the daily care at the end of the day. As the weeks go by after diagnosis, read up on the different choices, including pumps and continuous glucose monitors, and share the information with your teen. Encourage teens to share, regularly, about how their current method of care is affecting their day. For instance, if they find that a current plan demands they stop and eat a snack right in the middle of their varsity soccer match each day, let them know you can work as a team to find a solution. Then reach out to the medical team and ask them about options. With the many types of insulin and pumps available today, method of care can be tweaked and adapted to each person's unique lifestyle. For now, just be sure they know that there are many choices available, and you will help them find the method best for them at the current time, and work to change it when they feel it is needed.

While you will most likely seek out the input of others in the diabetes world, remember: each person with T1D is unique. For

> **Promote Flexibility**
>
> Newly diagnosed teens can feel they've been sentenced to a lifetime of rules and demands. While T1D is not going away, they do have choices in their daily care. Remind them of this regularly, and you may help them feel less "trapped."

some, pumps work great. For others, MDI is the best choice. Listen and learn, but in the end, remember no one can tell you what is best for your teen except your teen (and you). And at the end of the day, it does not matter which method is used, so long as one is used.

Transitioning Back into Daily Life

The transition back into daily life comes quickly, particularly if a teen is diagnosed during the school year. For some, it happens the day after the diagnosis. Others spend a few days in the hospital and then go back to life. One thing is usually always the same: this transition is more stressful for the parents than for the teen.

So how do you get them to jump back into "regular life"? Much as teens do not like plans, in the beginning, a good plan will help you all. For school, you are going to want a plan that involves blood glucose checks at certain times of the day and at least one visit to the school nurse at the start. (More on deciding when and how to use the nurse long term in chapter 7.) If your teen's school does not have a nurse (and this is more and more often the case with budget cuts today), you'll need to set up a plan for your teen to check and then check in with you via text, email, or phone call each time for the first weeks. Even with a nurse, for the first weeks, too, your teen should check in with you to report blood glucose readings as the day goes on. This is easy to do today, with cell phones and texting making it all a snap. You'll need to talk to your school about allowing your teen to text you (and talk to your teen about not misusing

> **Anything Is Doable**
>
> Parents may need to chant this to themselves, but also remind teens of it: there is almost nothing they cannot do with diabetes along. Whatever their hobbies, habits, and passions were, they will still remain.

that privilege). This will allow you to keep tabs and check in with the medical team when needed.

For after-school sports, the teen's coach(es) will need to be notified and given some basic education, as well as the school's trainer (if your school has one), who usually is on duty during sports practices each day. You and your teen will want to make clear to the coach that this diagnosis will have no impact on his or her ability to play the sport, and the coach should not worry about that. Teens should let coaches and trainers know that if they need to stop, they will speak up. Point out to the coach that many pro athletes play well with T1D, and your child will be no different.

What if there is no trainer on duty after school? This is not a reason to tell your teen that he or she cannot participate in sports and other events. Your teen's medical team has great experience with this. Work with them to come up with a plan for your teen and his or her activities. Remind teens that, in the beginning, it may mean some extra checks and extra hassle until you figure things out, but that they can and will take part in everything they enjoy. Diabetes will not stop them.

If your teen has an after-school job, the question of whether an employer needs to know that a person has T1D is a complicated one. Legally, it is none of their business. However, if your teen has already missed some work from a hospitalization, it may already be known. The best idea is probably for teens (on their own since if they are old enough to hold a job they are old enough to explain this without you) to explain that they will be carrying a meter, insulin, and glucose, but that it should not affect their ability to work in any way whatsoever. You may want your teen to run a bit higher at work and sports in the beginning as you figure out how things affect his or her blood sugar.

Is it okay to not tell an employer? Yes, it is. But usually, being upfront about the new change in your life puts people at ease and also alerts them in case there is a situation in which a teen needs help (which there most likely will not be). Still, better safe than sorry works.

If your teen is already driving, you'll need to have a serious talk and take some action before they can get behind the wheel again. Have them read chapter 9 of this book and then, together, discuss it and have your teen sign a driver's contract. Knowing how to handle driving with diabetes onboard is one of the most important responsibilities a teen has, and this should be taken quite seriously.

Setting Up Acceptable Communications

Communicating with your teen about just about anything is a snap, so why should a diagnosis of T1D make it any different? (Oh, we do like to make ourselves laugh sometimes.) One of the great ironies of having a teen diagnosed with T1D is that you've just stepped into a time in life when communication is key, but also a time in life when all your teen wants is be left alone.

This is a huge challenge for many. So how do you make it work without histrionics and battles? One way is by letting your teen know that all your constant communication could very well be temporary. Explain that for your educational sake as well as for his or her safety you are going to have to talk, text, speak, and share a lot over the coming months. Acknowledge that you realize this might seem like an imposition to them, but that your goal with all of this is to work to a place where you don't have to communicate as often.

So what do you need to communicate about? For the first months, it is your teen's blood sugars, activities, and, as much as is possible, food choices. It is imperative that teens know you are *not* looking for all this information to spy on them or even to call them to task for anything (And it is even more imperative that you *not* do that. Honesty is the best tool that can help your teen at this point). So, let's say your newly diagnosed teen is waiting for soccer practice to begin and a friend opens a bag of corn chips. She digs in, forgetting for the time being that she needs insulin to match those carbs. Later, she checks her blood sugar and it is high. What kind of communications should happen? In a perfect world, it would go like this:

- Teen reports (either by text, call, or in a logbook you share access to): *BG at 3 pm.: 342. Recall now that ate chips (did not count) at 2 and did not take insulin. Corrected with XX units.*

- Mom or Dad: *I see you realized the reason for your high and corrected. Nice job.* (Alternately, just take note and offer no comment.)

Note there was no "You ate chips without bolusing? You should know better!" Or, "Don't do that again!" Rather, the teen reported the facts and resolution, and the parent took note.

So what if your teen reports the same thing but with no correction mentioned? That would be a case in which the parent could say "You know, that will happen, and correcting later is a good idea. Next time you realize that, just check, correct, and move on."

You should expect, in the beginning, to review meter readings or a logbook each evening. This is because you and the medical team are, along with your teen, looking for trends and spikes as you figure out the best daily care plan for your child. If teens forget to check, simply make note and ask them if that is a hard time of day for them to check. Be open and willing to listen and to make adjustments.

There is language here that parents of the newly diagnosed teen need to understand. Consider these:

- There is no such thing as "good" or "bad" blood glucose readings. They are high or low, and just information to help with decisions moving forward. Often, people with T1D have no control over a high or a low, and, even if they do, it's a hard road that everyone has rough days on. Calling them good or bad assigns judgment to something that needs not be judged. Try to never call them good or bad. And when others say things like, "Is that good?" correct them politely and explain it's just high or low. Period.

- Regulation is a lousy word. Someone may ask you if your teen "regulated" yet. Explain to your teen and then to anyone who says it that T1D is about being in constant flux. Particularly while you are learning how to handle things and help your teen shoot for averages that make them feel good, there is no such thing as "regulation."

- Do not refer to your child as "a diabetic." Rather, say "a child with diabetes." Diabetes is just a part of the person your child is, not a label to put on them. Messaging that diabetes is something they have and not something they *are* is good subliminal support for your teen.

What if a teen is secretive about all this? In the beginning, that is not safe. You'll need to use your parental control to make sure they communicate with you until the time that your teen's medical team decides your child is ready to not share as much with you. Your teen needs to understand, too, that at this point it is absolutely imperative that all teachers, coaches, and others overseeing them know about the diabetes diagnosis. If teens are unwilling to share, let them know you will be sharing that information and that sharing it simply keeps them safe. If they don't like you for it, so be it. Just make sure you communicate with them how and why you are doing all this. Remind them: You are their defensive line. It might not be easy, but good communication will keep them safe and set them on a path toward good self-care in the future.

CHAPTER THREE

Diabetes and the Teen Diagnosed in Childhood

By the time my daughter hit the teen years, she'd been at diabetes for a good part of her life. I'd done my best to hold the reins for her, but in many ways, she had long ago started grabbing them herself. And sometimes I wasn't so sure that was a good thing. In hindsight, I know *it probably was not such a good thing—because by the time the teen years and the stubbornness that can come with it came along, I had a big job keeping control when I knew my daughter needed me to. We were at odds in some ways. She felt like this:* Gosh, I've been doing this forever. What the heck does anyone else know? *While I felt like this:* Everything is changing in her life. She needs guidance to figure it all out with diabetes in the picture. *There were disagreements, even battles.*

There were times when things did not go well. It tested our relationship, our trust in one another, and turned my hair gray (I'll blame the gray on that). We were, to put it simply, two people who loved one another but were completely at odds. It wasn't easy to find a middle ground, but eventually, we did. This chapter takes a look into the mind—and the heart—of the long-diagnosed teen. Hopefully it will help parents plan ahead, make adjustments, and not be afraid. It's not an easy time, but with patience and understanding, this too shall pass.

The teen years are a time of great change for the long-diagnosed teen and his or her parents. Both are used to a certain way of doing things. (Mom or dad oversees, child agrees. Oh, those were the days.) But as a child moves into the teen years, they move toward independence. Usually in life, parents celebrate this. After all, there's nothing like seeing your child sprout wings and fly. But with diabetes, it's all so different. First, parents worry. Second, teens resent. And that can be challenging. Thinking about it from both sides, having honest discussions, and working toward a place of cooperation and safety is the goal.

Teens Who Just Deal

There are long-diagnosed teens who do not struggle, who seem to just deal with their diabetes and not let it get to them. The secret? Might just be luck. Some people are more laid back, others less so. If your teen does not struggle, congrats—and skip this chapter!

Understanding it all from both points of view is far from easy. But the more you can do that, the better off your teen will be.

The Teen's Point of View

You are a fool and I know everything. The end.

Well, that's how they may think at this point. It's easy to see how they've come to that conclusion. First of all, the long-diagnosed teen has a lot of history with diabetes onboard. Many barely remember life without diabetes at all. They may have never gone to school without meters, blood check plans, and carb count stickers on their food. They've never stepped out onto a playing field without wondering if they will be high or low or if they drank enough Gatorade. They've attended countless medical appointments. They've gone back-to-school clothes shopping thinking—every time—"How will that work with my pump?" They've had to face challenges with aplomb and act mature in situations that many adults could barely handle.

So yes, they have a tendency of feeling like they know it all. And, in some ways, they do. But in the teen years, everything is changing. They see before them more freedom in their social lives, as friends are allowed to go to the movies and the mall and to walk downtown or go to the beach or the pool without parental supervision, and they want in. They see their friends talking more amongst themselves and less with parents, and they want in on that as well. The last thing they want to do, sometimes, is comb over a day of blood glucose readings and insulin decisions with mom or dad. They'd rather you just left them alone already.

The long-diagnosed teen, too, may be a bit sick of it all. (See chapters 11 and 12 for details on burnout and rebellion.) Carrying a meter, using a pump, counting those carbs—it's all just so draining on him or her. The long-diagnosed teen would like to wish it all away.

ON BEING DIAGNOSED EARLY FROM A TEEN PERSPECTIVE

Would it be better to be diagnosed as a small child, like I was, or later in life, like some other people I know were? It's a good question, and my answer to it has shifted as I've grown up. Having been diagnosed at the age of six, I have very few memories of what life was like without diabetes. I spent much of my life wishing I had been diagnosed at a later age. I thought that if I had not been diagnosed so young, perhaps I would not be as sick of diabetes as I felt sometimes. I thought, too, that perhaps if I'd been diagnosed later in life I'd be able to understand it better and accept it from the start. But recently, I have changed my opinion on this. After seeing one of my good friends from high school diagnosed at the age of eighteen, I realized that my not having any real memory of what life was like without diabetes was kind of a gift after all. Because, really, since I don't remember life without diabetes, I have nothing to miss.

I watched my friend struggle in ways that maybe were even more difficult than my struggles. Changing his entire life in the snap of a finger was not only difficult, it was emotionally upsetting. He struggled with acceptance for a long, long time (and in many ways, three years later, still is struggling). He was old enough to have developed a pattern of living, and I think a drastic change to that is hard when you really come to terms with what is going on. Plus, he was old enough to battle his parents on it, whereas I was not when I was diagnosed. To me it became clear that maybe earlier is better for a diagnosis (even though I hate using the world "better" for any diagnosis).

I believe that being diagnosed is a horrible thing for a child and the family at any age, and it was probably very upsetting for my parents when I was so little and facing all of this for the first time. But today, as I look back, I am happy that I wasn't old enough to really realize what was going on. That time was a traumatic time for me, and I do remember it being that way. However, I think that I was fortunate enough to be so young and dependent on my parents that they were there for everything I went through, and eventually as I got older, they taught me.

Sure, I went through burnout, but my feeling now is that all diabetes sufferers have their tough times. Had I not been diagnosed until I was a teen, those tough times might have hit before I or my parents had time to adapt to all of this.

So while the time I'd choose as the best time to be diagnosed is NEVER!, I think that today, with all I know, I might actually be glad I was diagnosed at a young age. While I had my struggles and I probably will have more, I was young enough for my parents to help imprint me with the basic understanding of what this life with type 1 diabetes is all about. I want a cure, but at least I know no other life than that with diabetes around. I have no life before diabetes to mourn, and in the end, that's one less thing to worry about.

Lauren Stanford

The Parents' Point of View

Your teen is like a toddler and needs you more than ever. Only you know every little thing about your teen's diabetes and can guide him or her through the teen years safely. The end.

That *is* how you think at this point, isn't it? And it's not all wrong. You have been closely linked to your child and diabetes for a long, long time now. When your child is sick, you are the one who keeps track of how the illness messes with his or her blood sugars. When they have soccer, you are the one who slips the extra glucose tabs and meter strips into the bag so there'll definitely be enough. (Or, as some teens would claim, enough to treat every kid with diabetes on the planet should they all show up at the game. But, you think, better safe than sorry.)

You are the one who has pored over your child's lab reports and tweaked basal rates, changed carb ratios, and generally been a 24/7 medical support team. The idea of the teen being able, at this point, to survive without you just seems daft.

In a perfect world, you'd like to keep children little. As much as you love seeing them making new friends, joining new clubs, and savoring their lives as teens, you want to protect. You want to hover. And you worry about them handling all this on their own.

What's a parent to do? What's a teen to do? When both are thinking in such different ways, those are tricky questions.

The "Model Patient" Shows Some Cracks

There are few parents who did not think when their child was still young that they'd really taught their child to be compliant and brave. And really, they had. Seeing a child deal with all they have to deal with when diabetes is onboard is really something to savor.

And if you told yourself—and even the world—that your child was a model patient and model person with diabetes when that child was, say, 10 or 11, you are not alone. If you celebrated when your child did his or her own shots, finger pricks, or site changes as if the child had won an Olympic event, you are also not alone. It's hard not to. But in hindsight, some parents often wonder if celebrating those things sends the wrong message to a child: that the child should be independent as soon as possible, when in fact, he or she still needs help and support. This celebrating can lead "model patients" to want to be just that for their parents: kids who can handle it all. Think of it this simple way—if you put your child with diabetes up on a pedestal, that child will have no way to go but down. Praise and support and thanks are all fine. But be careful about overdoing it. Subliminal suggestion can be dangerous.

For things can, and often do, change. Sometimes, the cracks begin to show and parents don't notice them. Teens, pushing for freedom but needing help, try to hide their struggle rather than share it. Some things to look for:

- **Missing checks more than a few times.** Okay, so all teens (and adults, for that matter) forget to check their blood sugar. After all, when you do something many times a day, it's easy to forget, or even decide to skip, one here and there. If you notice your teen has had more than a few misses or skips, even with a good reason ("My meter was left in my locker and I could not get there in time" ... "The battery died in my meter" ... "I was in too much of a rush"), you may want to consider the possibility that your teen is struggling a tiny bit and using excuses to hide it. Solution? Consider talking to your medical team about your teen having some say in how often he or she checks. It is possible that a frequency of checks they come up with (one that differs from your longtime practice) can be just as healthy. And if your teen makes the decisions along with his or her medical team and you are simply going along with it, your teen may feel a bit more "power and control" over this part of life with diabetes.

- **Skipped boluses.** These happen, too, because we are all only human. But if you see a trend toward this happening more often, your teen may be struggling. The same goes for unexplained highs (or explanations that make no sense). Patterns of these are often a visible hint that your teen needs help. Solution? Find a way to ensure your teen is taking insulin most of the time. You don't want to become "the enforcer" because there is enough challenge in your relationship now. Instead, if your teen is on a pump, tell them you need to stay up to speed on the technology and would like to review the pump setting regularly. There you can see a bolus history. If you don't like what you see, your challenge will be finding a way to react calmly (more on that in chapters 11 and 12). If your teen is on shots, watch them take at least one or two each day. If you see it going into them, you know it is happening.

- **Lying about it all.** This can be frustrating to parents, and many parents actually don't even notice the lying at first. Teens may choose to make up a blood glucose number and tell you that it's right. They may lie about how much insulin they've taken. It is important to understand that, while lying upsets all parents, you need to find a way for your teen to be able to be honest with you. Of course you can say that nothing he or she tells you would be punishable and that you understand a skipped bolus and/or glucose checks. But the teen is still going to be afraid of disappointing you. Rather, just don't ask.

Don't ask. It's simple: the meter and the pump and the pen and the insulin vial don't lie. Look at each once a day. Make note of what is going on or what is not going on, and then take it from there. Remember, your reaction will need to be a calm one. For instance:

"I notice you were not able to check all day today. Anything up? Oh, and here is your meter. Check now so you can correct if needed." It's a huge challenge for parents not to freak out at this. If you can do this early on, you may help your teen build a trust in you where they know they can be honest about the cracks that are showing in their diabetes care.

Suddenly Secretive

Remember when your child was an open book? When he or she wanted nothing more in life than to share experiences with you, the all-knowing and so-very-cool parent? Don't think it's diabetes making them secretive. One of the most classic teen movie scenes, after all, is the teen rushing through the house, slamming their bedroom door, and then talking, texting, Facebooking, Skypeing, or whatever, with someone—*anyone*—other than you. Suddenly, you feel out of the loop. Your teen is secretive.

It is one thing when you are just worrying about dating and grades and friendships and parties. Add diabetes to the mix and, again, it all becomes all the more stressful to the parent.

Because really, their daily diabetes care and how they handle things in life with diabetes along cannot be kept secret. So how is a parent to help a teen feel they have some privacy while still keeping tabs on all the diabetes information?

Open discussion with your teen, possibly along with the medical team, is a smart idea. Acknowledge that you understand your teen wants to have some privacy in their life. Tell them you completely understand that they don't want to share everything. But let them know that for the time being, you still need to play an active role in their diabetes care. Explain that it's not "spying," but rather supporting them as they move toward independence with diabetes. Then choose, as a team, some ways you can share information without being too "in their face."

With the advent of smartphones, there are more options for teens and parents to share diabetes information. And since teens are all about their handhelds, this may be a good idea. Ask your teen if they'd be willing to use an app that allows for the sharing of diabetes information during the day (and night). Point out that, with this, you might be able to train yourself to not speak with them in detail about their diabetes as often (a nice carrot for teens).

But the agreement has to be that they'll actually log in and share the information with you. (See chapter 4 for more ideas on tools that can help.)

The challenge to the teen, here, is to share honest and detailed information using the app. The challenge to the parent is to read it, review it, and only ask questions when truly necessary. For instance, if you begin to notice your teen is running high after lunch, discussing a possible increase in a lunch bolus is perfectly fine. However, discussing every number every day is not. If you decide to use an app, you'll need to remember to include cell

Watch Your Greeting

It's tempting for parents to say, "What were your numbers?" the moment a teen walks through the door after school or a day out. Don't do it. And don't ask two questions just to "fill space" until you get to asking about the diabetes. Teens don't like feeling like diabetes is the first thing you care about. Your words can make them feel that way, so work at not asking right away.

phone usage in your teen's school 504 plan (see chapter 7 for details). Likewise, you'll need to remind your teen not to abuse their permission to use their cell in school.

Using such a program does not mean you can depend on just it. Parents should set a hard and fast rule that the meter(s) in use needs to be left out for parents to look over once a day, and the pump (if being used) needs to be checked over as well. How do you do this without making your teen feel like they are under a dictatorship? Well, first, a home is not a democracy. But still, you don't want your teen to feel resentful. So with this agreement comes a promise from you: you won't ask them if they checked or took insulin. You'll simply "ask the meter or pump." Your challenge here, again, is to stay calm and not freak out. In fact, it might be better if you review the meter(s) and pump alone—which should not be a challenge since your teen is probably in their room Skypeing about you anyway. (You have to laugh.)

How do you handle it if and when your teen forgets or chooses not to log the information you feel you need to have? It's easy to get frustrated. To you, it just makes sense. Why would a person *not* want to make sure their health is fine and take all the steps toward that goal? But just think how hard some of the challenges we all face are (think sticking to a diet, quitting smoking, or adhering to a better workout schedule). We all flounder at times at things that are constant and challenging. Teens are certainly no different. So if and when your teen begins to not log what you need

Don't Forget Your Basic Tool Knowledge

It's easy to just let your teen run the pump or the meter or the insulin pen. After all, most times they want to just do it themselves. But here's a tip for parents of long-timers: If you no longer know how to operate every part of every tool your teen with diabetes uses for their care, you've let go too much. Keep up on how to work things, even if it's just to know how. It means if and when your teen needs you, you're ready. And it means you are paying attention.

to know, first of all, don't punish them. It's not fair, diabetes, and while you cannot use it to make excuses for your child, you also should not take away parts of their lives that have nothing to do with diabetes care. For instance: "You are grounded from Xbox because you did not log your information" does not work. However, "I'm sorry, but you failed to check at all overnight at that party. You need to show me you can keep track before I let you go to a party like that again. What plan do you have to show me you can?" works because they are directly related.

So if the app gets old and the teen stops using it, look for a new tool. Talk to your medical team about ideas other families are using. And most of all, ask your teen for input and ideas about how they can better communicate with you. If your teen says, "I'm sick of that app and would rather just text for a while," consider it. Any communication is good communication.

As for "faking" data for you, teens can and will do it from time to time. See chapter 11 for details.

Shifting Language and Expectations

As a parent, you have developed your own pattern of dealing with your child's diabetes. After all, this has had a major impact on your life, too. You've found a way to talk about it, discuss it, and work with it that works for you. But, being a parent means working hard to put your child's needs first. So as your teen changes how they want to be dealt with, so, too, must you adapt your way of discussing things with them and sometimes redefining what "success" means to you in this diabetes world. As always, your medical team can help you with this.

The first thing a parent needs to embrace is this: it does not help to get angry. True, it's hard to not be upset and angry sometimes. Diabetes stinks. And you are worried. And your teen's lack of ability to count their carbs or remember it all upsets you. But you need to find a way to work that out on your own time, not on your teen's time. Because chances are, they are just as frustrated as you are. Hearing you angry or disappointed is only going to upset them more. And while you cannot be expected to be Pollyanna (nor is that a good choice), you need to be one thing first and foremost: *calm*.

> **Sorry Works**
>
> If you do freak out or lose your cool, always remember to regroup and then apologize to your child. Doing so shows them that you are human, and that you know how to admit you were wrong and try to make it right. Great role modeling for how you want them to be.

This is no small feat. Some things you can do to work at a calm way to approach it all include:

- Remove the negatives from your vocabulary with your teen. Rather than say, "You did not check at lunch," say, "Can I help you find a better way or time to check before lunch?" Rather than say, "I cannot believe you didn't take your insulin again!" say, "Are you still happy with your pump (or shots if they are on shots)? Is it challenging to use them to take insulin at all?" Rephrase your worries to a question that shows you care, respect their opinions, and want them to succeed. Again: not easy.
- Don't make everything about diabetes. If you know your teen has done the sports drill they are going to do a million times, consider not discussing the diabetes end of it with them. Instead, sit back and let them work it out on their

own. Since they should be communicating with you and you are checking their meter and other devices, you'll know how they did. And when they do succeed, point it out. Pats on the back go far. And if they don't do well on a test or don't play well in a game, consider that it just might not have been their day. Suggesting blood sugars are the culprit every time can often upset and frustrate a teen. Even if you are thinking it in your head, don't bring it up unless they do.

• Threats don't work with teens. Telling them they might need a kidney transplant or have other complications does not work. First of all, teen minds simply do not consider the long term. We look at them and see grown-up (or nearly grown-up) bodies and assume there is a grown-up mind in there. But there is not. Teens have little ability to grasp the long term or consequences of actions long term. That's why speeding in cars and other dangerous activities are such an issue at this age. Second, this often backfires, as the long-time diagnosed teen hears it and thinks, "Well, I'm already doomed. May as well have fun!" And third, it is probably not true. Read up on the life span of people with diabetes today and the chances for complications. There is good news there and any such threat may be outdated.

Maintaining Control and Safety

At the end of the day, you just want your teen safe. Since long-diagnosed teens think they know it all, this can be hard for a parent to feel at peace with. But it's your job to keep them safe in life, so working toward a place where you are relatively at ease is as good for them as it is for you. Just make sure you are being reasonable in your goals.

In the end, if you can find a way to compromise (you don't get to actually do their blood glucose check yourself multiple times a day, but you do get access to the information; you don't get to sit a row behind them at the school assembly, but you do get to hear from them via text at some point during the long night), you can find a way to keep your teen safe, and, perhaps, even keep your heart beating steadily and slowly.

A Thought about Balance   *Meri Schumacher*

Balance—it is such a serene word, although infuriatingly complicated, too. We are told that balance is what we are aiming to achieve in life, yet there is nothing tangible about the word at all. If we are to achieve such a thing, wouldn't our benchmarks be biased? Certainly your idea of balance isn't the same as my idea of it. Yet here we are, all trying to achieve that elusive goal.

I often get asked how we balance having three children with type 1 diabetes with one child who does not. Frankly, it isn't easy to do. Obviously, there is a lot of weight on the one side of our scale. Diabetes gets a lot of attention in our house, as it is our normal. Is there even a way to balance our diabetic life with a life that is not about diabetes? Everything is affected by diabetes ... how can the scales be balanced when there is so much weight on one end?

To answer those questions, I would like to propose that maybe we are looking at this all wrong. Maybe we need to look at balancing more like a teeter-totter rather than a scale. On one side is our diabetic life, and on the other is everything that does not have to do with diabetes. Envisioning that teeter-totter in my head, I can see that our diabetic life spends a lot of time with its tail on the ground. The reality is, we don't get to feel the wind in our hair very often. But when we do ... man, there is no better feeling! Feeling the whisk into the air as our life finds normalcy is thrilling. It isn't fun being grounded with the weight of stress and responsibility. We need to be lifted once in a while and be granted the views that can only come from relieving ourselves from the heaviness. That is why our family spends most of its time loading up the other side of the teeter-totter with the little things. We try to find things that bring us joy, and as we do, the weight of those little things adds up. We try to normal our way through our days, putting in the work, but not necessarily letting all that work weigh us down. The more we count our blessings, the lighter our diabetic life tends to be.

Sure, our idea of balance is going up and down, up and down. Some might argue that we could find better balance in the center of the teeter-totter. If we sat right in the middle, gathering all the weight from either end, surely we'd be able to achieve the true definition of balance. No up. No down. Just flatness.

Honestly, though ... what fun would that be?

I'd much rather enjoy the ride.

Meri Schumacher is the mother to four boys, three who have type 1 diabetes. Her children were diagnosed at the ages of 8 months, 2 years, and 5 years. In 2012 Meri also lost her husband to cancer. Muddling her way through all the emotional phases diabetes and grief have to offer, she knows the worry that sits with us like an old friend, because it is her friend, too. Her motto is: Try your best. Love your best. Hope your best. You can't do better than your best. Meri blogs her ongoing story at www.ourdiabeticlife.com.

CHAPTER FOUR

Tools of the Trade and Their Use during the Teen Years

At the risk of sounding like your old Aunt Bessie who constantly reminds you she had to walk barefoot in the snow uphill both ways to get to school each day, I need to share something here: When my daughter was first diagnosed years and years ago, I had to walk barefoot in the snow uphill both ways to get her diabetes supplies, and those supplies were nothing like the supplies you have to choose from today.

Okay, I'm exaggerating, but only a little. Parents dealing with a child with diabetes today need to realize that much has changed, even in just the past 15 years. When my daughter was a child, there was no such thing as rapid-acting insulin. Nor was there such a thing as non-peaking long-acting *insulin. (Lantus was not approved for use in children until April 2000.) Pumps were available, but it was almost unheard of for a child under 16 to be on one in most cities. (We had one endocrinologist tell us, "You can drive a pump when you can drive a car." We were happy to prove him wrong, as my daughter became one of the first young children in our state to pump insulin.) Meal plans were rigid and restrictive, and schedules were tight. Diabetes is far from simple today, but it's also far from the restricted, complicated way it was just a decade or so ago.*

Today, there are more and more great tools available, and it delights me to see my daughter, as a young adult, considering them, learning about them, and yes, using them. To me, the increase in tools and in ways to handle diabetes on a daily basis means more flexibility, more changes to feel "in the driver's seat," and more ways to shake things up in a good way through the teen years.

I hope this chapter educates you and encourages you to learn, along with your teen, about the many choices you have on this journey. And the story by Dr. Aaron Kowalski, one of the premier researchers overseeing the advent of new diabetes tools in this world (and a person with type 1 diabetes), should inspire you. Maybe in a few years you'll be able to say you walked both ways barefoot through the snow compared to what's out there. Here's hoping.

You already know that your diabetes toolbox is a complicated one, possibly more complicated than any carpenter, artist, or lineman's toolbox could ever be. Who does not remember how shocking it was the first time you got all those prescriptions filled and looked at all the paraphernalia you now needed to add to your parenting quiver? The great thing today is that there are more and more options and choices for people with diabetes. From a plethora of insulin choices, to a variety of pumps, to cool meters, to new technology, there is a lot to consider. And while it's great to find tools that work and settle in with them, with teens sometimes change can be a good thing. Knowing what is out there and what it could do for you is good information to have on hand. And letting teens know they can tweak and choose when it comes to their daily care might hand them a bit of the feeling of control they crave. It is important to remember here that, thankfully, the diabetes-tool landscape is ever-changing. By the time this book hits your hands, there could be even more great tools available.

Insulin Choices

It wasn't so long ago (the 1980s) that most people with type 1 diabetes took one shot a day and hoped for the best. There were those who experimented with multiple daily injections, but they were few and far between. In fact, since insulin was first invented circa 1923, not much changed for decades and decades. This meant it was nearly impossible to have any kind of true "target range" for diabetes care, and it meant lows and highs were a given.

Thankfully, that is no longer the case. We now have blood glucose meters to check blood sugars regularly. We have A1C tests to find our three-month range and give us a better idea of what is going on long term. And while insulin is still a medication that's

Insulin Peaks and Timing Chart

Here is a great chart to see how different insulin works in the body:
www.diabetesnet.com/about-diabetes/insulin/insulin-action-time

difficult to manage in an exact way, the many choices one has now means we can get better and better at it. Medical teams work with patients to find a combination that works for them. It is important here to remember that diabetes mantra: your diabetes may vary. A combination of insulins that works well for one person may not be best for another. And conversely, if a certain combination spelled disaster for you, that does not mean it will as well for another.

Pumps versus MDI

It has almost become like the breast-feeding question, fraught with judgment: "Your child *is* pumping, right?" While insulin pumps are relatively new to the diabetes world (two decades ago you'd have had to search hard to find someone on one), they've leapt quickly to the forefront of care.

And for good reason. Pumping insulin can offer a person with diabetes more freedom, more precision, and less stress on a management basis. But they can be tricky, too: pumps need to be paid attention to quite closely. So what are the benefits of pumping, and what are the benefits of MDI? Both offer their own, and while many like to claim pumping is the only right choice, in reality, with the many types of insulin available today, the decision of pump versus MDI is mostly a personal one.

Pumping Pros and Cons

The pros of pumping are many. First of all, since the pump delivers a "basal" insulin dose to the body 24/7, people with diabetes can tweak how much of that basal they are getting at any time. In theory, a well-planned basal profile should allow a person with T1D to go 24 hours without eating while staying in an acceptable glucose range. This means that if a person tends to go low in the late afternoon, he or she can adjust the pump to

cut back on insulin just before that time. Or those who experience the pre-sunrise spike many have known as "dawn phenomenon" can dial up their basal to automatically give them more insulin to combat that occurrence.

Pumping makes bolusing for food or highs easy, too. Since your insulin is right in your pump and is delivered to your body via a tube under your skin, bolusing means simply adding up the carb count and pushing some buttons on the pump to deliver it. Most pumps even have programs that know how many carbs are in certain foods, or that allow you to input certain meals you like to eat. You dial them up, you push a button, and your insulin dose is done.

Pumping can also mean carrying around less, but in a perfect world, it should not. Since the "rules of pumping" advise that any highs are corrected via a shot, anyone on a pump should be carrying around a backup shot and insulin just in case. Pumpers also need to always have on hand a backup site change in case their pump sites go bad. Still, you won't need to be married to having a vial of insulin and syringes with you at all times.

There are some red flags to pumping, too. First, since an insulin pump delivers only rapid-acting insulin, should a pump fail, or should there be a problem (such as a clogged site or a site falling out without notice), the risk of developing ketoacidosis is higher than on shots. This is because on MDI, your "basal" or "background" insulin is administered by shot and at one time, offering a "safety net" in the case of highs. In other words, once that shot is in you, it stays in you for 24 hours. On a pump, there is no long acting. This means a person on a pump must be vigilant about checking blood sugars and detecting highs, since all the insulin going into your body, be it via a basal pattern or a bolus, is rapid acting. That means that at any given time, you are three to four hours away from no insulin going into your body, in the case of a pump or site problem.

Pump users also need to rotate infusion sites as well. The site, which is the connection where the pump sends insulin into the body, can be placed in any area of the body with fatty tissue. But over time, overused sites can build up scar tissue and not work as well. Overuse of a site area can also cause "atrophy," a denting in of the skin. While rotating shots is important, rotating site locations is very important as well.

Pumps are also, for the most part, visible. Some people do not like the visible reminder of their diabetes attached to them all the time. While there are many ways to wear a pump that keeps it out of sight (we share some later in this chapter), there are teens who just don't like it. But for the most part, teens are happy to trade having to wear a device for the freedom they find it brings them.

For a teen, pumping can mean the ability to tweak insulin doses to help with sports days and no-sports days, longer and shorter busy days, and special activi-

> ## Which Pump Is Best for Your Teen?
>
> Today, there are more pump choices than ever before, with many new models and brands on the market. Which is best for your teen? A great spot to check out all the models is this web page: www.children withdiabetes.com/pumps/

ties. It can mean being able to simply pull out a pump and bolus, rather than deal with using needles and insulin vials in school or at work. It can mean being able to take the pump off and stop delivery if they are going low or heading into a big game. On the con side, the pump means responsibility for a teen. It is up to them to push those buttons and to make sure they are paying attention to the pump as it functions, as well as not losing it (this happens!).

MDI Pros and Cons

Multiple daily injections are still the way a majority of people treat their diabetes, although pump use is increasing daily. MDI used to mean a set schedule and lack of freedom, but with today's insulins patients can work with their medical teams to come up with an MDI plan that still gives them much freedom.

The benefit of MDIs is that people can give themselves a shot of their long-acting and know, for sure, that their body has insulin in it for at least those 24 hours. With rapid-acting combined, MDIs mean that diabetes sufferers can have flexibility of when to eat or when not to eat, since they simply need to add up their carbs and administer a shot any time they need to.

Insulin pens have made MDIs friendlier as well. Pens look like, well, pens. Almost all types of insulin can be administered via pen now, which means a person can pull one out just about anywhere and not get the looks one might get with a syringe and vial. Pens also mean a person can dial up his or her dose, instead of having to pull insulin out of a vial and into a syringe (which means worrying about things like air bubbles). Pens make carrying around your MDI supplies easier and less bulky.

The con of MDIs is that you don't have as much flexibility in your basal insulin. Since you have to pick a dose and stick with it, you cannot tweak it by the hour as you can on a pump. However, with things like split doses, you can have some flexibility. Another con is the amount of material you need to carry around with you.

For teens, MDI is sometimes preferable because they are tired of, or not interested in, having something attached to their bodies. A pump is a constant reminder of diabetes, and some just need to get away from that. Some teens find that MDI forces them to comply more as well, since taking shots tends to be more of a routine.

"Pumpcations"

So, what about the idea of switching back and forth from pumps to MDI, and then to pumps again? This is becoming more and more popular, and could be a great strategy to help a teen get through these rough years when burnout always seems to be hovering on the horizon.

Most parents feel that once children switch over to pumping, they never want to go back to shots. In fact, for parents who get used to pumping, the idea of MDI can be frightening. Pump advocates believe there is little chance of having tight control on MDI. But in reality, you can have tight control on either.

Usually, if teens are looking for a pump break, they have a reason. It might be they are tired of having a piece of machinery attached to them 24/7. It could be they've become lackadaisical about their diabetes care and realize they are not giving the pump the time and attention it requires. It could be they are feeling the need to begin to separate from their parents, and since their parents know pump care inside and out, they wonder if shots might help them begin that process. It could be they are just feeling the need for a change. Whatever the reason a teen asks for a pump break (or "pumpcation," as we are calling it here), parents need to listen.

Taking a break from pumping does not have to be a big deal. In some ways, it can even be helpful. Since it's always a good idea to be up-to-date on MDI and how to manage with it (in case of a pump problem or another kind of emergency), taking a break from time to time will force your child—and you—to brush up on MDI basics. (It's easy to forget them over time. And if your child has been pumping for years, you may never have experienced MDI with Lantus or Levemir.) A pump break can also give those pump sites a short rest, something that can be good for them over the long haul.

Summers Off

Some teens like to take the summer off from pumping. With bathing suits and summer clothes and lots of trips to the beach or the pool, pumps can get in the way a little more than usual. If your teen wants to, let him or her take a summer off from pumping.

But most of all, the pumpcation might just give teens something they crave more than they can express: a sense of control and choice in a world that seldom gives them that. You cannot give your teen a vacation from diabetes. Even if you offer to take over all the care, it's still the teen's body living with it and experiencing it. That can be frustrating and grinding for a teen, particularly one who has been facing diabetes for a long time. If taking a break from the pump makes him or her feel in control, then why not?

Some teens report that either switching off the pump for a while or going back on it gives them a new chance to focus and forces them to pay more attention to their daily care. Teens get complacent, be it toward their longtime pumps or their longtime MDI plans. A switch can help them re-focus.

It's also okay to go off the pump for a special occasion such as the prom or some other event for which the teen might not want the pump around. In all these cases, you'll want to talk to your teen's medical team to come up with a plan for that time.

CGMs and Teens

The first continuous glucose monitor available to the public hit the shelves in 2006. Marketed by Medtronic, it was a larger device that was attached via insertion and then a wire to the pump site. Within months, Medtronic had replaced it with a much smaller model with no additional attachment wires. Shortly after that, Dexcom hit the market.

Today, more and more companies are dipping into the CGM field, and all are modernizing the product, making new models more accurate, smaller, and easier to use. True, there is a long way to go before CGMs are seamless, and everyone is looking forward to the day when they truly interact with pumps (making those pumps "smart pumps" that not only determine what a person's blood glucose is, but also react to it to treat the person with ease).

When the first inpatient clinical trials were done on CGMs around 2008, an interesting finding became clear: the patient group who fared the worst on CGMs in trials was teens. This was because they did not—or could not—adhere to the stringent rules of the trials. Ironically, with hormones and burnout and the challenges of the teen years, teens might just be the age group of people with diabetes who can benefit most from them.

So, Is a CGM Right for Your Teen?

Here are some important things to know. First, you do not have to be on an insulin pump to use a CGM. Even brands like Medtronic, which are paired with a pump, have a non-pump option. Second, CGMs do not have to be used 24/7, although for the best results, using them at all times is a good idea.

CGMs work like this: a small wire probe is inserted under the skin (in much the same way a pump site is inserted). This, depending on the brand, is either connected to a transmitter or already attached to one. Then, depending on the brand, it checks blood glucose every five minutes and transmits that number to a pump or to a receiver device. People with diabetes can then look and see not only a recent blood sugar reading, but a graph and charts that show where they've been, and with some brands, arrows that show if they are trending up or trending downward. Alarms can be set for low and high blood sugar readings, which means you'd be notified whenever you got to one of those two numbers.

Finger pricks are still necessary. First, you need to calibrate the meter, usually twice a day. Second, CGMs are still not always 100 percent accurate, so most advise you to still check a few times a day, or any time you have a reading that seems questionable to you.

For teens, a CGM can mean more information at a time when their body and hormones are playing games with insulin absorption and use. It can also mean gathering more information and data for sports, work shifts, and other issues they may want to understand more about to handle best. And when used correctly, it can mean more information for parents and caregivers to download and study—without having to pick the brain of the teen that much.

The con of a CGM for most teens is another device attached to the body. Some teens don't like the idea of that, and balk at using them. One solution for parents who want that information from a CGM might be to use one a few days at a time or a week or so each month, and then to use the information gleaned from that to made adjustments or dose changes.

Goodbye Meter? Not So Fast

CGMs are not, at this time, meant to replace blood glucose meters or even checks. In fact, you'll have to check a few times a day at least to calibrate the meter and keep it on track.

The Future of CGMs and More

The real hope is to move toward a time when CGMs and pumps work in tandem. The idea of the "artificial pancreas" is to create a CGM that not only communicates with a pump, but understands how insulin works in the user's body and then tells the pump to give more or less insulin based on the trends it detects while in use. In Europe there is already a system on the market with "glucose suspend" that, when blood sugars are low, stops the flow of insulin from the pump into the body until the person's blood sugars come back into a higher range.

There are also human clinical tests on smart pumps, or apps, going on in a few hospitals across the country. In the summer of 2013, researchers hope to do their first out-of-hospital human trials on smart pumps, possibly at diabetes camps.

The idea of taking part in a clinical trial is appealing to some teens, not so exciting to others. The upside of volunteering for one (and there are many upsides) includes getting to see a new product before it hits the market, getting to see how new technology works before the rest of the world does, getting a chance to have some top researchers focus on your diabetes for a few days and longer, knowing you are making a difference in the world, and more. Usually, participants are paid a stipend as well. And of course, they are seen as heroes.

There's another benefit, too, particularly from taking part in an app trial. Said one teen who spent her college vacation week as an inpatient at Yale on the app, which meant she did not have to check her blood sugar, count her carbs, consider exercise impact, or even think of what she was doing or eating for a week, "It was the best vacation I ever had in my life." The idea of being "free" of diabetes even in a hospital setting is often welcomed by teens.

The flip side is simple: it's hard work and a sacrifice. Clinical trials are demanding, and you are checked and tested and looked at and relooked at many times over the course of them. For some teens, an extended trial can be almost too much to adhere to. And inpatient trials mean giving up time in their busy lives.

Clinical Trial Participation

To find out how you or your teen can take part in a clinical trial, go to www.trials .jdrf.org and sign up for information.

Smart pumps or the app may be the next best thing to come down the pike, when and if they do come. And while smart pumps or the app are certainly not a cure, for teens particularly, the idea of taking some of the burden of diabetes off their shoulders is a valid one that many hope to see come true soon. For many, a better tool that eases the burden is a nice goal to reach along the way as the world works toward a cure.

Managing Meters

One meter, two meters, three meters, or more? It's a question parents and teens have to consider and decide on. It's not easy to work off more than one meter, and sometimes it's not the best idea. But it's also frustrating for teens to have to always remember to have a meter with them.

In addition, deciding which meter used to be simple: there were so few that you'd simply go with the one your medical team suggested. But with the modernization (and exponential increase in cool factor) of meters, there are many to consider. Since there are so many, with new ones coming on the market regularly, we won't mention all the brands here, but will focus more on what they do and how and why to use them. For a good, up-to-date list of meters and reviews of them, go to www.childrenwithdiabetes.com. CWD keeps the list well updated as new meters hit the market.

So your first thought is: what kind of meter do you want your teen to use? Here, there are so many choices now, with cool add-ons they can do. While you'll have to ask your medical team about prescription approval for strips, most who have coverage for any meter can get coverage for any other meter. There are, of course, exceptions. But if there is a meter your teen is jazzed about and your insurance says no, most endocrinologists know how to work the system and get it covered.

There are lots of interesting new twists in meters now. From downloadable with the push of a button (and the plugging in of a cord—or not!), to interfacing with an iPhone, to tracking trends and then suggesting what you should focus on, meters are getting smarter and smarter. And there are real benefits to that not just for teens but for parents. Some meters (like the iBGStar from Sanofi, which connects to the iPhone) have apps as well, which parents and teens can both load onto their smartphones to keep track of things. Many, too, have easy ways for users to send their results to parents and/or their medical teams via e-mail. It really does make sharing and checking in easier when you have a modern meter.

However, teens are not always happy about sharing this information. While the meter may do a great job of gathering and sharing, that also means your teen may feel "spied on." It should be your goal, when a teen shares this information, not to stress over every number. (Remember, *any* number is a "good" number because the teen checked. There is no such thing as

Sometimes New and Cool Makes All the Difference

For teens who are tired of checking and a bit burned out on diabetes, sometimes a new tool like a cool new meter is motivational. If your teen is sick of checking, consider shopping for a new meter. It might just help a bit.

good or bad in a blood glucose value when reviewing meter data.) It should also be your goal not to discuss it daily. Respect that your teen is being cooperative, and try to keep input to a minimum, which may mean a new "what's necessary" for you. While your teen still absolutely needs you, you also need to find a way to continue to slowly move toward independence. Meter review and discussion can be a time when teens balk at your input. Manage it with kid gloves.

How Many Meters?

In a perfect world, your teen would work from one meter and only one meter at all times. This makes it easier for everyone—for you and the medical team to see data and trends, for you to manage strip prescription refills, and for the teen to keep track of. Since most teens carry book bags in school, it should be simple enough for them to carry it with them at all times during and after school (and even if they go to the nurse's office to check, they can pull that meter out and use it). For boys, who don't tend to carry "man purses," this can be a challenge outside of the school day.

Since there is a lot to tuck into a pocket (meter, strips, backup insulin, etc.), many parents of teen boys find they don't mind those small backpacks made of nylon that close with a string and loop over your shoulders. Others use ziplock plastic bags (two usually) that can be tucked in pockets.

The challenge with one meter is simple: teens are forgetful (well, we all are, really). And as important as it might seem to someone on the outside of this diabetes world to remember to bring along your life-sustaining supplies and equipment, because our goal is to raise our teens to live their lives first and bring diabetes along second, things can be forgotten.

For many people with diabetes, a machine that could do what their pancreas did before diabetes would be a dream come true. It seems so simple. We have insulin pumps, we have continuous glucose sensors, and we sent a man to the moon more than forty years ago! So, why don't we have one yet and why is it so important?

My family has been dealing with diabetes for longer than thirty-five years. In 1977, my younger brother Steve was just 3 years old when, like a bolt out of the blue, he was diagnosed with "juvenile diabetes," as type 1 was called at the time. In 1984, at the age of 13, I was also diagnosed with type 1 diabetes. Two of the six children in our family, a family with no prior history of any diabetes, were now faced with a lifetime of replacing the insulin our bodies could no longer make. Unfortunately, at that time, replacing insulin required multiple injections a day and was an incredibly imprecise science. At the time of my diagnosis, we had just begun to monitor blood sugar and still used insulins that were harvested from cows and pigs. Diabetes treatment was really still in the Dark Ages.

Raising a family with two kids with diabetes in the house wasn't easy. I give my parents a ton of credit. One thing that they always told us was that we could do any-thing our friends without diabetes could do—and more! That said, we all knew how that would take more work and it would not be easy. And, even with two very smart and dedicated parents, managing diabetes at that time was so very hard. Some of my most vivid memories growing up are of hypoglycemic seizures, ambulances outside our home, and how incredibly scary diabetes could be.

We've come a long way. Today, I'm fortunate to be on the front line of diabetes re-search leading the Treatment Therapies research program at the JDRF. Treatments have evolved quite a bit since our family first faced diabetes. We have insulin pumps that eliminate insulin shots and provide more freedom to people with diabetes. We have continuous glucose monitors that provide real-time glucose levels 24 hours a day and alarms if blood sugar levels are too high or too low. We have better insulins. But the person with diabetes and their family still must bear an incredible burden in trying to replicate what evolution took millions of years to perfect—regulating blood sugar levels. Even today we know from research that people who stick their fingers more than 10 times a day—trying to aggressively manage their diabetes—spend less than 30 percent of the day in the "normal" blood sugar range. At JDRF, our goal is to cure diabetes and to walk away, back to a life without the disease. While we work to that goal, the focus of the JDRF treatment program that I work on is to accelerate the development of tools that improve blood sugars and reduce the burden of managing the disease.

That brings us back to the Artificial Pancreas. How is it that we could send a man to the moon forty years ago, can fly airplanes with hundreds of people on them primarily by autopilot, but can't deliver insulin automatically? The issue is that insulin can be a very dangerous drug. Too much insulin at the wrong time can cause life-threatening low blood sugar. We must create systems that are safe. It can be done. In the late 1970s, research into the artificial pancreas had begun and the results were very promising. Using these first artificial pancreas systems, blood sugars could be normalized. The problem—the first artificial pancreas was the size of a refrigerator! This does not meet our criteria for success—while glucose is improved, there would be a lot of burden toting a fridge around everywhere you go. Today, miniaturization of these systems is a reality. The same insulin pumps that many people with diabetes use every day will soon become automated; initially some of the time and eventually most of the time. This will meet both of our goals—reducing the amount of work that people with diabetes and their loved ones will need to do while improving their blood sugar control. Research around the world is showing that this works, and now companies are developing these systems so that people with diabetes will benefit in the near future.

The future for diabetes treatments, as we drive toward a cure, is bright. When our family first faced diabetes, we were told of the incredible challenges we'd face and the high likelihood that we'd face the terrible complications of the disease. Today, nearly 35 years later, both my brother and I have been fortunate to live without complications, to have wonderful families and successful jobs. I've run 11 marathons, even qualifying for the Boston Marathon! Having diabetes doesn't mean we need to have any limits! In the near future, treatment will become even better—easing much more of the burden of diabetes and keeping us healthier. The dream of the first artificial pancreas systems will soon become a reality.

Aaron Kowalski, PhD, oversees JDRF-funded research aimed at accelerating the delivery of therapies that will help keep people healthy while living with type 1 diabetes, minimizing their risk for developing diabetes complications, as well as therapies that will help those who have developed diabetic complications. Dr. Kowalski is an internationally recognized expert in the area of diabetes technologies and has been a leader of JDRF's Artificial Pancreas Project, a multimillion dollar initiative that began in 2005 to accelerate the progress toward a closed-loop automated insulin-delivery system.

That's why you need backup. And while it is always best to work from the same brand of meter (for strip supply reasons more than for anything else), here it is okay to save money and simply purchase (or get for free) a less-expensive one and store it where your teen might need it—with the school nurse, in the bottom of a sports bag, or anywhere else you can think of one might be needed in a pinch.

The danger of backup meters is that you can lose track of your teen's numbers and that teens can claim to have done checks they may not have done. (See chapters 11 and 12 for why teens may do just that, as well as for signs to look for to know that may be happening.) A good idea for the school nurse meter is to ask the nurse to email you when a check is done there with the number and the time of day it was done. You do not need to ask your teen to do this or tell him or her it is happening. It will just help keep up to date.

Free Backup Meters?

Since the meter companies make their money on your use of their strips, it is often easy to get a free backup meter (or two) from them. Contact your customer support line or attend a diabetes expo and see if you can score a free backup or two.

As for your teen telling you, "I did check on my other meter," remember, you don't have to argue. You can just "ask the meter." If your teen has a backup meter or two, take a look at them once a week. And as always, it is your challenge to not react in a negative way if you don't see what you expect or what you were told was there. The information—or lack thereof—serves as details to help you move forward and know what is going on (or not going on) in your teen's life with diabetes away from you.

Ketone Meters

Not so long ago, your only option for checking ketones was urine strips. And while every home (and school nurse's office) should still have a supply of the urine strips, a ketone meter is a must for any family raising a teen with diabetes.

First and foremost, the meter is a current look at ketone levels. Strips, because they check via urine processed by the body, run about two hours behind blood levels. Many families find they can better manage illnesses and ketones with a meter and its up-to-the-minute readings.

Ketone meters are not that expensive (and many of the companies offering them will send you a free one via their web sites). The strips, however, can be a challenge to get covered. Talk to your endo team, for they recognize this and can help you. And even if you can only get a smaller number covered, you can use the ketone meter and backup with the urine strips if needed.

Overall, the device and insulin choices available today are remarkable, and the range of choices is only growing. Knowing what is out there and keeping up to speed on what is coming down the pike can help teens not only manage things better, but understand that in a world that seems to control them, they do have choices.

And that can be empowering.

CHAPTER FIVE

Diabetes, the Teen, and Family Dynamics

Way back when my daughter was newly diagnosed and still in the hospital, I took my older daughter, then ten, for a walk outside the hospital walls. I wanted her to know that I had not forgotten her and that for a while, at least, things were going to be topsy-turvy.

As we walked along, hand in hand, I shared with her how things were now and made a vow for the future.

"For a while, you are going to feel like all you hear is 'Lauren, Lauren, Lauren. Diabetes, diabetes, diabetes'," I said. "And there's nothing I can do about that. But in time—maybe a few months—it will all settle in, and things will be back to 'normal'. (I wish I'd said we will settle into a 'new normal.') I need to ask you to be patient and *understanding while we adjust to all this."*

Of course Leigh said yes. She's that kind of kid. Now I have to laugh at the vow because, 16 years later, Lauren's diabetes still holds a prominent role in our family.

I wish I could say I'd treated my two girls absolutely equally, but I have not. We love them equally, but they each have unique needs. And that has not always come out "even." A diabetes diagnosis completely shifts family dynamics. For my family, it meant absolutely still doing all the things we ever did (ski trips, beach days, spontaneous dinners out, just plain life, laughing, and enjoying things), but always with that added layer of "the diabetes decisions."

We did our best to thrive despite it all, and we did. My husband and I are still married. My older daughter is currently getting lots of attention as we plan her wedding. Lauren is off at college learning to deal with diabetes on her own.

But it wasn't easy. I believe that protecting the core that is your family is as important to a successful future with diabetes onboard as, well, as blood glucose control. It's easy to let a difficult diagnosis and complicated life pull you apart. But joy—and a wonderful sense of accomplishment— come with using these feelings to pull you closer together. No easy task. Here's hoping this chapter helps you do just that.

It doesn't take long in life with T1D onboard to realize that diabetes is very much a "family disease." While only one child usually has it (of course there are cases of more than one child and even a parent and child), diabetes has a way of seeping into every nook and cranny of a family's life. You can see it in a physical way: drawers and cabinets that once held snacks or crafting supplies are now dedicated to diabetes supplies. Ketone strips stand at alert on every bathroom sink. Used test strips pop up seemingly everywhere.

You can see it in an emotional way, too. Whether a teen is newly diagnosed or has been at this for a long time, "what about the diabetes" prefaces almost every decision a family makes as a unit. Planning vacations, tweaking family budgets, managing sick days, and just plain living every day with diabetes means a part of the parents'—and each family member's brain—is always on diabetes.

For families with more recently diagnosed teens, this can mean an upheaval the likes of which they've never felt before. For long-diagnosed teens, this can mean a level of burnout from other family members ("Aren't we used to all this yet? Hasn't it gone away?") that can be crushing and disappointing.

But it can be managed. While it's not easy to smooth out a family life with a teen with diabetes around, it can be done. Focusing on it as a family and working on honestly shared feelings and, yes, sometimes just sucking it up, can all help a family stay unified, strong, and maybe even all the better for this.

The Sibling Factor

Teen siblings bicker with one another. They fight over sweatshirts. They complain you give more to the other than to them. The words

"It's not fair!" ring through homes of teens often. With diabetes along, all that can be amplified. So how does a parent handle things when one sibling is a teen with diabetes?

First, you have to remember that with diabetes, you have no choice but to spend added time on a child. Just managing prescriptions, insurance companies, and medical appointment calendars alone is a job. When you consider you also have to make sure your teen with diabetes is taking care at school, at sports, behind the wheel, and even at home under your nose, the idea of giving equal time to a sibling seems impossible. But it's not completely impossible.

The first thing you need to do is understand how the sibling of the teen with diabetes is feeling. Some common feelings include:

- **Guilt.** Siblings may not say it out loud, but if they don't have T1D, they often harbor guilt about being the one who did not get it. So, too, can they feel guilt about being jealous of the added attention their sibling with diabetes gets. It is important for parents to keep ahead of this. Remind your child without diabetes that it's not his or her fault and that he or she should not feel guilty. And let the teen without diabetes know that sometimes you are secretly frustrated by all that diabetes demands of your family. Knowing you, too, can feel frustration can help that teen not feel guilty about being sick of it sometimes.
- **Fear.** Siblings without diabetes live with a lot of fear—fear they might get T1D themselves. Fear something terrible will happen to their sibling with T1D. Fear of the future ("Will he/she be there to be an auntie/uncle to my child one day?" "Will something terrible happen to them?") It's important to educate your children about the future and about diabetes in general. Our world is different now. The

chances of severe complications are greatly diminished. Your child will hear other things. Remember to let the sibling learn and embrace the very high chance of a bright future for the other sibling despite diabetes. As for the fear of getting T1D, share the statistics with your teen that there is only a slight chance of that teen developing T1D, barely more than for a person without a sibling with diabetes. Help your teen see that the chances are slim, and that he or she needs to live life well and not stress about what the future might or might not bring.

> **TrialNet: Is It Right for Your Child without Diabetes?**
>
> TrialNet is a program that gathers blood samples and information on direct family members of a person with T1D and uses them in two ways: for research toward causes and a cure and to pinpoint the possibility of someone developing T1D. Whether it is right for your family or not is a personal decision. Families who do take part are heralded as heroes, and well they should be. The information gathered is helping. But if a sibling absolutely does not want to take part, you need to listen to that teen. It's his or her body and his or her choice.

- **Jealousy.** Even when a sibling with T1D is being rushed off to the hospital, the sibling without can be left feeling jealous. It's hard when a lot of a parent's attention has to go to one child. Things like family walk teams, other fundraisers, support groups, and even, in some cases, media attention can focus a lot of energy on the child with diabetes. Most families know enough to try to include siblings, but usually siblings are just left out of the spotlight. What is a parent to do? Make an effort to celebrate things in the life of your child without diabetes. Science fairs. Soccer games. An art show. Brag on it, savor it, take the teen out to a special dinner to celebrate a little more than some other families might. It's often surprising to teens with diabetes when the other sibling gets attention: they see how it feels to be the one looking in, which can be good for them, too.

- **Anger.** Siblings can just plain get sick of it. It's okay for them to lash out about it from time to time—but not directly against you or your teen with diabetes. In this instance, you need to help your child without diabetes learn to focus their anger and work through it, using the same tactics you would with your child with diabetes. Admit that it's lousy. Tell them you get it. Then encourage them to take some quiet time, do some writing, calm down, and refocus. It's a good life lesson they can get from dealing with diabetes in the house. You also need to quietly explain to your child with diabetes that a sibling may have some of these feelings, particularly anger, because the anger may manifest itself against the child with diabetes. Helping the teen understand that a sibling might be struggling, too, might help him or her better deal with any anger that comes along.

So what if your teen with diabetes uses the situation to "lord it" over the child without diabetes? It's not unusual for teens in general to try to manipulate a household to their own liking. Having T1D can be a powerful tool in doing just that, and it must be stopped. True, you have no choice but to focus a lot of your attention on diabetes. But you also can make sure that does not get out of line. As an example, what if both your children have a sporting event at the same time? Would you always choose to attend the one your teen with diabetes is playing in, because "you have to be there"? The answer needs to be no. First off, teens can learn to manage their diabetes well in sporting events without you there every time (see chapter 7). Second, if there are two parents involved, you can adopt the "divide and conquer" strategy that many parents of siblings (even without diabetes) adopt: trade off and each attend a different child's event, switching each time. It might even be a good practice to sometimes err on the side of attending the event for the sibling without diabetes.

What about when highs or lows get in the way of a plan? True, there are going to be times when you just have to stop everything and treat for a while. You need to remind the sibling without diabetes that were he or she to get sick—a stomach bug, strep, or another illness—you'd take the same course of action. But it's also a good practice to keep on going whenever you can. Let's say you planned on going to the big mall that's an hour away. All of a sudden your teen with diabetes is a bit high. Can you bring along what you need and check along the way? This not only shows that diabetes can be woven into life even when it's playing games with you, it also shows children with diabetes that they can power on through some challenges. It shows your child without diabetes that when you do say "we have to stop," it's for good

> **Playing the "D-Card"**
>
> If your teen tries to "play the diabetes card," you need to nip it in the bud. Parents often report that teens suddenly feel low when chore time comes, or claim to feel they might be going high when a family event they are not interested in comes along. Showing them that diabetes does not stop them ("I'm sorry you are low. Treat the low and then go about your chores.") will show them that playing the D-card does not work at home or in life, a good lesson.

> **Celebrate the Sibling, Too**
>
> Many families celebrate "di-aversaries," anniversaries of the day a child was diagnosed. Remember to include siblings in the celebration. A small gift, a family dinner, a cake with each of their names on it; anything to remind the siblings that they, too, have been victorious over another year with T1D in the house.

reason, since you don't automatically cancel all plans based on a blood sugar reading or two. Flexibility—showing your children how to maintain it even with diabetes along can help them see that life does go on … even with some bumps.

At the end of the day, parents have to find balance in an unbalanced world. With teens and siblings, this is not easy even without diabetes onboard. Remember to remind your children of that. And sometimes, it's okay to just say it like it is: "Right now, you are right. It does not feel 'fair.' But kiddo: that's life."

Extended Family and the Teen with Diabetes

Whether your teen is new to diabetes or a long-timer, extended family and their understanding (and acceptance) can be a slippery slope.

For the newly diagnosed, many family members may simply not understand what T1D is. It's up to you to educate them. Ask them to read up on some easy web sites (such as jdrf.org and its "life with diabetes" section, or *www.diabetes.org* and its type 1 section). Purchase them a basic book on type 1 and kids (it all translates to teens, after all) and encourage them to ask questions.

But don't expect them to completely get it. So many people confuse T1D with type 2. They assume your teen cannot eat sugar or sweets, and think they know what the future holds (and in some cases feel obligated to share that misinformation with you, your teen, and anyone else who will listen).

Support for Extended Family

When little children are diagnosed, parents often think to send grandparents, aunts, uncles, and others to support programs or educational groups. This is just as useful when a teen has diabetes. Even with a longer-diagnosed teen, encouraging relatives to attend a support program can open their eyes, re-educate them, and better equip them to support your teen well.

A Diabetes Diagnosis and Siblings   Regina Shirley, RD, LDN

When I was growing up as the baby of the family, my two older sisters had their moments of smothering me with attention and then switching to jealous outbursts at all the attention I was getting. I was always the carefree spirit among the three of us, and my overly confident and charismatic disposition often annoyed them, I'm sure. When I was diagnosed with T1D at age 9, my sisters were 13 and 14. Those ages are tough enough—being girls, going through puberty—without having your youngest sister bring a chronic disease into the mix. The usual drama—fighting over a sweater or sharing a room with my middle sister or not liking the same music—became forgotten in the house of eggshells that everyone had to walk on. All of a sudden, they had to change their lives. They had to find new places to hide cookies or help me at school when the kids started asking questions about my disease, and most of all they had to grow up way too fast to support my quickly crumbling parents.

Diabetes goes though the rough stages right along with the teenager who lives with it. The toughest part for teens is ever admitting you still need your family for support. My parents kept me and my diabetes at a manageable distance, to where they could see us both, but not intrude unless they saw any damage being done. They let me learn my lessons and have never let me forget that they are always there, even if it's just to let me complain. The best advice I can give to a parent or sibling of a teen with diabetes is to let him or her live life, but don't leave the bread-crumbs far behind in case the teen needs to be reminded that there is a familiar path nearby ... and keep that up even when the teen is well beyond needing you.

My family is and always has been supportive, in the best way they know how. Whenever I leave my sister's house after visiting with my nephews and start my hour-long drive home, she piles my purse with granola bars, fruit snacks, and juice boxes meant for toddlers. She mumbles, "Oh, there's only 8 grams of sugar in that, but that's enough, right?" She is always obsessed with whether I have eaten lunch and often forces me to eat the leftover mac and cheese that my nephews pushed aside (I gladly accept because mac and cheese is one of my vices). How would I even begin to explain to my sister or my mother that I haven't been on NPH in over 12 years, and that I don't need to eat much for lunch or any lunch at all if I don't feel like it? The details are irrelevant, because they care enough to try. So for all those years I have felt that I did my sisters an injustice by stealing my mother's time away from them, they never stopped caring or loving me and worrying about my well-being, so I let them worry.

As the years have gone by, my sisters and I have traded places on needing my parents more than the other one, so I don't feel so guilty much anymore. While I took my mother away from my sisters for a good part of their teenage years, more recently, my sisters have needed my mother more in their lives than I have as an adult, and so she has once again taken her place as their protector, advocate, and caregiver. My sisters have never come out and said that they blame me or my diabetes for affecting their growing up, but I will always carry that guilt a little bit in the back of my mind. As a soon-to-be mother, I also recognize that as a parent it is okay to lift children up when they are down, but there is a fine line between advocating for a child who needs it and constantly walking around with an apparent black cloud above your family for all to see. There are positive ways to make diabetes a part of the family dynamic, and there are destructive ways as well. My parents and my sisters did the best they could, and it has taught me more than anything how to be a better sister, daughter, and mother myself.

Regina Shirley has lived with T1D for more than 22 years. She is a registered dietitian working as a diabetes and nutrition consultant. Regina runs a diabetes and nutrition blog www.ServingUpDiabetes.com, which serves as an informative resource to inspire health, wellness, and a unique perspective on real life with T1D. Regina is an active volunteer for the Bay State Chapter of JDRF and is a past keynote speaker for the Fund a Cure Gala in New Hampshire

For long-time diagnosed teens, extended family may not understand why they are not "regulated" (using that word we don't want to use ever), or why your family is not "used to it all yet."

Both cases can be hurtful to the teen with diabetes. Teens, even if they don't show it, crave support, understanding, compassion, and love from all of their extended family. They may not understand how a family member can be ignorant, and get frustrated and hurt by them. The best thing you can do is communicate openly with those family members and encourage and enable them to be a positive voice in your teen's life, instead of one that upsets, disappoints, or frightens your teen.

You'll need to remind relatives, as your teen grows, that he or she can eat almost anything, so long as it is covered by insulin, and that there is no need to comment on what your teen chooses to eat or not eat. Ask them to refrain from comments like "Should you be having that?"

And what about the relatives who are afraid to include your teen with diabetes in sleepovers, camping trips, and other events? This can be upsetting to teens who see cousins doing things they'd like to join. Reach out to your family members and ask them what they fear, and then educate that fear right out of them. Just as you learned, family members can learn that teens with diabetes can really do anything, and that relatives who support unrestricted ambitions are helping a teen grow into a confident, independent adult with diabetes.

In the end, some relatives are never going to get it and never come around. All you can do is use that as a lesson for your teen with diabetes and your other children. Point out to them how you've all tried to get them to come around and they have not. Encourage them to remember to never be that person, and to always be open to learning how to help others in life.

Single Parents and the Teen with Diabetes

It's hard enough to stay on the same page with a spouse when you live under the same roof and share the same goals. For divorced or never-married parents of a teen with diabetes, all this can be triply challenging. And teens know it. Don't be surprised if your teen tries to play you against one another, or chooses to head off to stay with one parent to avoid the rules and diabetes demands of another. What are parents to do? As impossible as it may seem, you have to find a way to work together. If you have a relatively respectful relationship, this won't be as challenging, although it will have some bumps as any parenting relationship does. And if you are not on speaking terms, you are going to have to find a way to communicate and cooperate.

Your first step should be letting your teen know, with both of you in the room, that you will be communicating and sharing about your teen's entire life—including his or her diabetes. Set the goal of putting personal feelings aside, for the sake of your child's health. In fact, is it probably a good idea for both you and the other parent to attend diabetes appointments together from time to time (along with any other stepparents who are in the picture). In time, this won't be necessary (and you don't want to crowd the room), but at the very least the doctor's follow-up letters should go to all parents so all can stay informed.

> **Communication Is a Must**
>
> You don't want to have to grill your child every time he or she gets home on what went on and how things went at the other parent's home. Instead, set up an online logbook for the parents to share and agree to log into it, even if it seems tedious. This way your questions will be answered without having to involve your child.

Here is a key for parents on both sides to remember: there are many ways to care for diabetes. While you may feel your way is right and your ex-spouse's is wrong, in the end, we all have our own ways. So long as your child's medical team is onboard and supportive, you may have to allow for some differences in daily care while your child is at the other parent's home. While this may be hard to swallow, consider this: married couples often face the same challenge. It's not unique to divorced or unmarried teams.

And what if you feel your child is in danger at the other parent's home? Your first step should be to discuss it with someone on your child's medical team, be that the endo, certified diabetes educator (CDE), or social worker. You need to do so with honesty and an open mind. They can help you see if you are correct and help you take action, or see that your child is fine there and help you learn to deal with it.

You'll also need to ask your medical team to help you get enough supplies via prescription to stock both houses. While you cannot get double, you should be able to get enough that you can store backups at each home. Choose one home (the primary residence) for the majority of supplies to be stored. Expect some things to have to go back and forth with your child, but plan for backups so they are in place in case of an emergency.

It's easy to want to just cut the other parent out, but with diabetes, the more team a teen can see working in harmony, the better. It's the ultimate challenge, perhaps, but one worth trying for.

Parents as a Role Model

You don't have to have diabetes to be a role model for your child. The teen years, with hormonal weight gain and temptations in life, are the perfect time to begin new positive lifetime practices. Parents should look at their own lives and see if they, too, can work on self-improvement in an open and shared way, one that will role model for their teen the best way to live a healthy life. In other words, if you are overweight, this is a good time to focus on better eating and exercising. If you are sedentary, it's a great time to pick up a new activity or sport that gets you moving more.

So let's say your teen with diabetes is struggling with not wanting to do blood glucose checks, or to count carbs and cover with insulin when eating. You, too, have not been watching what you eat. So you share with your teen that you will be planning your meals better, counting carbs, and focusing on staying on track.

This can be a shared experience for the two of you. Of course you are not going to be perfect, and through this, you can show your teen how to not give up, how to know that one off day does not ruin a lifetime. You can also show teens honesty. If you fall flat on your face with your plan, share that with your teen. Ask teens for advice (which will make them think about how they handle their own challenges). Show them that a fall does not mean you've failed. It just means you have to get up and start again.

You may want to consider taking up an activity together as well. Cycling is great for a parent and teen; so is running. The popular Couch-to-5K program available for free online is a great way for a parent and child to work toward a goal. Choose a fun 5K in your area that's six months off. Start up the program together and then run it as a family. You'll not only get in better shape, you'll introduce your teen to goal setting, planning, and a new way to work off steam and keep blood sugars down. You can even choose a reward once you've accomplished your 5K, bike ride, or whatever your goal is. A spa day, a trip to a favorite restaurant, or whatever makes you happy. Set the goal as a family and do it as a team. As you work toward your goal, help your teen learn to manage diabetes, but let the teen lead you on that quest. While you are the parent and it is your job to make sure he or she gets it right, encourage your teen to read up on how to best manage blood sugars during the activity. Have teens consider their performance when higher or lower. Talk about it, and let them lead as you supervise. This, after all, will be what they do in life as an adult.

Through this, it is important for a parent to role model honesty, too. If you struggle, don't hide it. If you "cheat" on a diet, don't hide it. It's better to show your child that everyone struggles, and that it is what you do after that struggle that defines the person you are. Many teens feel once they've fallen short with their diabetes care a few times, trying any more is pointless. We know this is not the case. Show them just that with your own life.

You may want to consider a challenging new sport that you all begin as a family as well. Snowboarding, skiing, tennis, and any other sports that people can do for their entire lives are great choices. You'll learn as a unit and grow in it together. You'll build memories. And in the end, teens with diabetes will have another sport to keep them fit as an adult with diabetes. Not a bad reward for working on something new.

CHAPTER SIX

Diabetes and Friendships in the Teen Years

I can remember the moment as if it were right now. *Lauren was just at the age where we'd allow her—along with friends—to wander past the pool area of our private beach club and out onto the sand beach without parents. It wasn't far: if parents stood at the club gate or up on the deck, they could spot their children and every move they were making.*

But to the kids—little as they were—it felt like a great adventure. They'd make "forts" in the giant barrier rocks; they'd watch the tourists all covered in oil. They loved going over there sans parents.

Of course, we had that added layer of diabetes to consider. Lauren was still pretty little, but she had something more valuable than the most advanced glucose meter or the smartest CGM in her "pocket." Even at a tiny age, she had friends who "got it."

So one day, the girls were all over the beach doing whatever, and suddenly, two of them came running from the beach in a way that just screamed danger. Everyone looked up from their books or knitting or laps or tennis and watched as Kelsey and Breezy ran directly to me.

"It's Lauren!" Kelsey said, grabbing my hand and dragging me along, somewhat breathlessly. "She's low. She felt it but we didn't want to risk her walking back here yet. You have to HURRY!" Breezy was grabbing my other hand, pulling me along.

Over at the beach, Lauren was laid out like a princess. Her good friend Emily had tucked a towel under her head and was stroking her face, as if to soothe her. Liz was squatting next to her, holding a juice box to her lips.

"We got it from someone on the beach," Kelsey explained. "We had glucose tabs but we wanted to make sure!"

Lauren looked up at me, and I could swear she winked. She was fine. Yes, she'd been low. She later told me that she probably could have just had a glucose tab or two or walked back over to me, but when she said she felt low, her group of friends sprang into action. And she said she just knew she had to let them help her. "So they'd know they could,

Mom." It all made sense. Did I mention this group of girls was all of eight years old at the time?

I had known it before, but I realized it that day: Lauren was blessed with an amazing group of friends. From the day she was diagnosed (when they were all kindergartners or around that age), they not only accepted that one of their tribe had something new to deal with, but learned all they could and stepped up as protectors, listeners, providers, and guards. Oh, and most of all, friends.

They've stuck with her over the years, too. Our glory years of the JDRF Walk, when our team was huge and brought in a ton, came largely thanks to that group of friends and their families (and our adult friends as well). As Lauren grew and wanted more freedom, I had an ace in my own pocket: at least one of those close, smart, caring friends was almost always with her. It was like sending along a spare pair of my own eyes, and it helped me say "absolutely" many times in her life. Like the first time she went to a movie without parents along. Or the first time bowling. Or the long, long bike rides that the gang used to take (that always included a "snack stop" at the Dunkin at our local hospital).

She added some friends as she grew up, too. In high school, I could always count on Ben and Sully to have Lauren's back. Lauren would tell me how, when she was *in a phase of just not wanting to check, Ben would check his own blood sugar first, so she wouldn't feel alone. Both are off serving and protecting now, and you have no idea how my heart soared when I got a donation to my Ride to Cure Diabetes from Sully, who is away on active duty. Now those are some friends who stick. And who get it. And how about her prom date and still good friend Ryan? Ryan withstood me showing him how to use a glucacon, and then came up with his own amazing plan: every few hours, all night long, he'd text Lauren. She'd feel her phone buzz from inside her cute clutch and—as any teen would do—immediately open it to see who was texting her. It was Ryan, and it said, "Your meter is right here. Now check." Lauren said it was so cool how he helped her take care that night in a sensitive and private way. They are friends to this day, and I'm happy about that.*

Even when Lauren went off to college, I knew the girls and guys were always checking in on her via Facebook, texting, or Facetime. I'm not sure I've ever come out and said it to them but I say it now: Without you kids, I'm not sure I'd have been able to raise Lauren as such an independent, self-assured, worldly young woman with diabetes. So thank you.

Which makes me wonder about what it means when parents are afraid to let their child go off and hang out with other kids. I totally get it: it's our job to worry and to protect. But I wonder if by easing children into playgroups and playtime and time just alone with friends as they grow, we might be doing one of the best services we can do for our children with diabetes.

Because with mommy right there, kids are never going to step up and take charge. But with a little breathing space and a decent amount of education, they are going to do just that.

When Lauren went off to college I feared a lot, and a big part of it was not having Holly, Kelsey, Breezy, Emily, and Liz along to watch closely, to grab a juice box from a total stranger, and, yes, to tuck a towel under her head and stroke her cheek if she just needed soothing.

But Lauren had learned well from her dear friends, and soon I was hearing new names. Like Deanna. And the Katies. And more Laurens. And Nick. Now, she still has that same group of great friends whom I call the "since the sandbox gang," but she has another quiver of pals to count on as well. One that I have to laugh about is Nick. Nick is more than just a friend, you see. And here's a funny thing about that: when he asks her to remember her Lantus, it's caring. When I ask, it's nagging. I'm fine with that, by the way.

Friends who get it. Freedom to let them take charge. Now there's a diabetes tool every person needs. This chapter talks about how to use that tool in the best way for your teen.

Friends—and the social world created by them—may very well be *the* most motivating factor in the life of the average teen. What they say means so much more than what mom or dad says. What they think is worth poring over for hours, even days. What friends want to do becomes a must. It's a powerful force and bond.

For the teen with diabetes, forging, building, keeping, and protecting friendships can take on a whole new meaning. Even for teens who grew up with diabetes onboard, these years can be a time of confusion about how to share and when to share, since so many new friendships begin in the teen years (with a move to a new school, changes in hobbies, sports choices, and kids working toward what they are really interested in, many new friends are made in these years).

The best thing teens can do, of course, is have their friends know about their diabetes, understand it, and be compassionate and protective because of it. But remember: the last thing most teens want to be is different. Or weak. And in their minds, sometimes they might feel like diabetes makes them seem that way.

Helping teens know how to build strong friendships based on honesty is like adding another strong tool to their diabetes toolbox. If you can help them understand why it's all worth it, they might just see the light and build special friendships that not only make them happy, but keep them safe and you—the parent—more relaxed.

Friends and the Newly Diagnosed Teen

When a person is diagnosed with diabetes as a young child, enlisting the understanding and support of friends is relatively simple. Mom and/or dad goes into school and reads a story (usually about a bear with diabetes who tells all his bear friends at school all about it). Then children bravely show their friends in school their meter, their insulin, and describe their day. The kids rally. They go home and tell their parents all about it. In almost no time, most kids—and families—get it and support it.

But you cannot really go into your teen's class and read a story. Or go in at all. In fact, other than the sharing of the news and details with the school administration and teachers, the job of sharing is now up to your teen.

So how are parents to convince teens that sharing their diagnosis and what it means for them to have diabetes with their friends is the best option? It may take some doing. First things first (and when diagnosed, the medical team should tell your teen this as well): sharing and explaining make it all easier and make it less of a big deal.

Getting to Know Diabetes Dinner

Throw your teen a "getting to know diabetes dinner" to which they can invite a group of close friends. There, your teen can show them the devices he or she uses and give the basics on what it means in their daily teen life. And you can serve pizza and ice cream, putting to rest from the start that "Wait, you can't eat that, can you?" vibe most newly diagnosed teens get.

If your newly diagnosed teen was hospitalized, that may make breaking the ice easier. In most schools and communities, particularly with social media, news travels fast. If your child was hospitalized, chances are most people know something is up. That does not mean they understand it, though. So you'll need to explain to your teen that most people don't understand the difference between type 1 and type 2 diabetes. You'll want to arm them with some basic talking points (not just for friends but for everyone!) so they can explain it in a way that makes sense to the uninitiated.

Do not expect your teen to want to go to school or out with friends and announce, "Hey! I have diabetes now!" But encourage them to find a way to "seamlessly" add it into their day with their friends. For instance, even if your teen does not have to check, he or she may want to in front of a group of friends when with them, at least once. Suggest that your teen nonchalantly pull the meter out and instead of letting friends gawk or be confused, say something like "Yeah, so this is my glucose meter. Watch what I have to do now—it's kind of a pain, but I have to do it a few times a day so you guys may as well get used to it." Questions are bound to follow, and with luck, the next time the meter is pulled out, those friends won't be as surprised.

What if your teen refuses to tell any of his or her friends? Secrecy is not an optimal plan in life with diabetes, and the sooner your teen learns that, the better. It is okay, in this case, to go behind a teen's back a bit and talk to the parents of the teen's closest friends. Let them know that your teen is feeling strange and worried about sharing, and that it really is best for them to share. Their friends, if they are good friends, should be willing to listen to "clever and polite" ways to bring the subject up with your teen. Help them know what to say, such as "I know you were diagnosed with type 1 diabetes, but I don't know what that means. Can you tell me—and tell me how I can make this easier on you?" Having the others ask might help your teen open up a bit.

Sharing with Friends for the Long-Diagnosed Teen

Teens make new friends. So even if your child has had diabetes for a handful of years or more, the "telling" thing can become an issue in these years. Kids who once just matter-of-factly told anyone might suddenly not be as forward with it. This is usually because, like most teens, they want to fit in and not feel different.

As your teen makes new friends, you may want to ask, in a nonconfrontational way, if anything has been shared about diabetes with them. Expect to get a huffy non-response, some stomping feet, and possibly a slammed bedroom door. Hope to get an answer, even if the answer is "Why would I?" Your teen needs to be reminded that as always has been the case, it is better for people to know than to wonder. You as a parent need to feel your teen is comfortable with diabetes in the open because, logistically, it keeps him or her safer. Since teens are often not at home, they should be doing a fair amount of checking and bolusing out in the world and with their friends, including their new friends. Not wanting to share might lead them to hiding those actions or worse, avoiding them. The better you can get your teen to learn that most kids are completely fine with the information and won't judge, the better off your teen will be.

So obviously, you don't expect your teen to say, "Hi, I'm Sue and I have diabetes!" the moment she meets someone. And let your child know that. But suggest that they just simply explain in a few words when they pull out their meter, a pump, or a needle to use it.

In some ways, though, it's a good thing if your teen is not thinking about diabetes first when he or she makes new friends. You want your teen to live as "normal" a life as possible, and not thinking of diabetes first when building a new friendship could very well be a sign of that balance. Just help your teen to remember that the sooner someone knows (and again, this can be as simple as doing a check in front of a new friend or pulling out a pump to bolus and then matter-of-factly explaining), the sooner it is not a big deal. Even teens who have had diabetes for years may need to be reminded of that.

> ### A Telling a Friend Writing Project
>
> Teens have to complete writing projects all the time for school. Suggest, as a way for them to help your local diabetes support group, that they write a "how to" on how and when to tell friends about their diabetes. Ask them to do it with a child a couple of years younger than the teen who is facing the same challenge. Not only could this be of service, it will help your teen think through the issue—without nagging.

Enlisting Friends as Helpers and Supporters

Teens can—and should—realize that their friends can be powerful tools to help them through these teen years with diabetes, and in many ways.

First off, even if they won't admit it, teens want and need support and backup with all this. While they may complain endlessly and call even the smallest comment a nag, deep down they are thankful you care. The same goes for their friends. Teens with diabetes will just feel better—more relaxed, comfortable, and at ease—with friends who understand diabetes and have their backs.

So how can one enlist friends to help? By doing it both passively and aggressively. Teens need to be shown that sometimes friends just need to be clued in. If you can and your teen will listen, show through example how friends can help one another. For instance, perhaps you have an adult friend with a food allergy. Tell your teen with diabetes how that friend supplied you with a list of ingredients to avoid when you cook for her, and that now she knows she can visit your home as a guest and be safe. Tell them how good that makes you feel.

While avoiding foods is not an issue for teens with diabetes (a bigger issue is friends knowing they *can* eat most foods by knowing the carb count and then taking insulin for it), if you can find a similar situation like this to share with your teen you might help the teen in wanting to enlist friends.

The best thing teens can do for their friends is help them understand what type 1 is, what it means in their daily life, what they worry about, and what they need support on. Here are some helpful things for friends of your teen with diabetes to know. (If you could get your teen or the parents of your teen's friends to share this with them, it could help.)

- Teens with diabetes can eat almost anything; it just takes work. Sometimes, though, it is just easier not to have pizza right after you had ice cream right after you had high-sugar coffee drinks. The best social situations are those that might not include food after food after food just because it's a lot of counting and checking and insulin-taking.
- Teens with diabetes should always check their blood sugar before driving a car. There is no special danger to teens with diabetes driving a car as long as they do this. Friends should consider it as vital as seatbelts (which by the way are vital!). It's okay to be supportive in this—and say something like "Well, let me set up your meter before we go! Copilot duties!"
- Teens with diabetes should always have fast-acting glucose readily available. Want to be an amazing friend? Go to the pharmacy or supermarket and buy a tube of glucose tablets and tuck them away in your car or your bag. Some day when your friend with diabetes is low, pull them out and say, "Hey! I've got you covered!" It's a little thing that could mean a lot.
- Teens with diabetes may have to carry more stuff than you do. For boys in particular, this can be a challenge. Why not start carrying some kind of satchel or bag like your friend has to carry as well? If all your close friends carried similar bags, it would not be as big a deal to your friend with diabetes.
- Read all you can about type 1 diabetes and what it is so you understand it, but do not lecture like you know more. Simply have it in your head so you truly get it.
- Just tell them you care every once and a while. It means a lot.

The Nonsocial or Shy Teen with Diabetes

Not all teens are outgoing, and the parent of the shy teen knows this is not something you can change. Shyness is a part of a person's makeup. Shyness can get in the way of sharing anything about diabetes with friends or acquaintances. Parents of shy teens will need to let teens know and understand that the sooner people know about their diabetes, the less of an issue it will be.

Let shy teens know they don't have to shout it from the rooftops or become a public speaker for the cause, but they do have to be open to anyone they keep close to them that they do have diabetes. It's a safety issue, to state it simply. But also let them know they don't have to share more than the basics if that is their preference. What it is and what to do if they need help ("grab my cell and just autodial my mom if I say I need help") are enough basics to keep friends in the loop without forcing a shy teen to open up too much.

Making a Difference

Teens with diabetes can also enlist their friends to make a difference in the treatment and cure world. Most, if not all, teens have required community service hours. Some sports teams are even required to perform one community service act per person per sports season. Of course teens with diabetes are going to feel awkward suggesting that their friends or their team do something for them in particular.

But it's okay here for parents or friends to plant the seed. Find a local walk for a charity that your teen with diabetes cares about, and see if you can get his or her friends to want to take part. Even if they simply run a car wash or raise a little bit of money, taking part in it will mean learning more about type 1 diabetes, understanding what needs to be done in the world to help people with type 1 diabetes, and taking action in a fun way that shows support.

If there is no kind of walk or event close to your area, look for an online program teens would feel passionate about and suggest they do something locally to support that program. While this may feel "selfish" to your teen, point out that by showing friends how to help, your teen is helping kids learn how to be philanthropic and how to help make the world a better place: both qualities anyone would want future adults to have.

And by all means, make it fun. Let the teens add a "party" feel to it all. If you can, hire a bus to transport them to and from an event or host a small party at your home once the event is over. Not only will you have helped your teen and his or her friends bond more, they will have helped the world. There are a list of suggested charities and programs in the appendix of this book.

When Friends Annoy

Friends, like parents, can become "nags" in the eyes of the teen. As with parents, it's because they care. Teens may tell you that some friends have upset them in one way or another, and you need to know how to help them let their friends know what to say and when to say it. But so, too, you need to help teens understand that some of that behavior from their friends may come from true concern. Here are some examples of teen friends.

- **The Know-It-All.** This friend either has a relative with diabetes or has read up on it a bit and begins to lecture your teen on what he or she does well, does poorly, and needs to change. Sometimes, the teen is one who is looking to go into medicine and therefore believes he or she is ready to be your child's doctor as well. They might say things like

"Whoa, not a good food choice there!" or "I read that with more exercise you can cut back on your insulin." It's annoying enough to a parent. To a teen, particularly one who understands diabetes and its implications, it's sometimes too much to handle. So what's a teen to do? The best thing you can advise teens to do is sit the friend down, alone, and say that it's all too much. The teen has let his or her friend know that the concern is really appreciated, but that every person with diabetes is unique. It's not easy for teens to communicate with one another this way, but if your teen is willing to, it may help. It is important that you, the parent, do not get involved. Your teen is at an age when he or she should handle these things on one's own. And you may want to tell your teen that adults say those things to you, too, and sometimes you just nod and say "Whatever."

- **The Overly Caring Friend.** This is the friend who really, really wants your teen to be safe. Secretly, you'd like to buy them a pony. But just as it's not the best thing for you to question every move your teen with diabetes makes, neither is it a good idea for a friend to be constantly saying "Have you checked?" "Are you low?" "Are you high?" and all the rest. What's a teen to do? In a perfect world, teens tell friends like this that while they know they care, it can get to be a bit much and feel more like parenting than friendship. If teens are willing, they should give such friends a "role" in it all so they can feel like they are helping. Some ideas include: carrying a carb counting book or having one on their phone and being willing to count a teen's carbs at school lunch or out to eat; or setting up your teen's meter when he or she is about to use it. Sometimes these little acts can help both sides of the situation.

- **The Unsupportive Friend.** This friend is the one who says, "Oh come on, just forget about it for now. You are being way too worried." It is simply not the place of another teen to tell your child this. Of course, your teen may love that and buy into it. If you notice your teen's self-management is off when he or she is with certain friends, you may want to pay close attention and find a way to help your teen realize it's up to teens, not their friends, to decide how to care for themselves.

> **Warning: Don't "Use" Your Teen's Friends**
>
> It's tempting to use friends to do what you want to do, but know you should not. Do not ask friends (and particularly romantic interests) to ask your child to check or peek at a meter and report back to you. This is unfair, as tempting as it is.

"Diabetes World Friends" and How to Find Them

There is nothing like a friend who truly gets it, and who never needs explanation or advice on what is going on with your diabetes. Thankfully, in most cases, there are not a ton of kids with diabetes in close proximity to you. So it may involve some searching out to find them. If your teen is newer to diabetes, they may give you pushback on this. But in the end, it is almost always worth the effort.

A great place for teens to find friends who get it is diabetes camp. Diabetes camps can be found in most states and even in other countries. Because they are staffed for the most part by folks who grew up with diabetes (and always have medical staff on site), you can be relatively sure your teen will be safe while there.

What happens there is often called magical. Teens bond in a

way that they simply cannot even with their own families, because they are surrounded by other teens living exactly the same life. And while some people say they don't want their teens to go to diabetes camp because they don't want them to "feel different," the opposite is true at camp. Because everyone there has diabetes, things like checking, taking insulin, and treating highs and lows simply become commonplace and almost beside the point. The friendships that form there last a lifetime. And even though camp ends, thanks to smartphones and the Internet, the kids stay close. A list of associations and some top camps is included in the appendix of this book.

There are events you can attend as a family, too, that help kids make friends. Talk to your local pediatric hospital about having your teen volunteer at an event for younger children, or attend a teen or family event. You may have to drag them kicking and screaming, but they might just make some friends. Other options include advocacy and fundraising for diabetes programs. You can read more about advocacy and events in chapter 16.

"Friends for Life" is an internationally respected event that takes place in Orlando, Florida, every July. This program brings more than 3,000 families with children with diabetes to one place. Teens have their own mini program within the program that includes classes, a semi-formal dance, a day trip to Disney World without parents (!!), and lots of bonding. It's well worth considering as a way to help teens find some lifelong friends who understand what they are going through.

In the end, helping teens help their friends as well as find friends who have diabetes may be one of the best tools you can give them. Until the cure, they will need to know how to surround themselves with supportive people and help those who surround them become just that. With that, they'll be safe, cared for, and understood. And that's what any parent would call a win.

There's No Place Like Camp — Kelly Kunik

You want your teens to experience some instant D-bonding while simultaneously learning how to own their diabetes? Of course you do! Send them to diabetes camp.

I'm serious—take a deep breath and let them experience a few weeks with other teens and tweens living the same D-life they are. And I know whereof I speak because I experienced instant D-bonding at the now defunct (but never forgotten and always close to my heart) Camp Firefly in lovely Spring Mountain, Pennsylvania. Yes, for three years in a row (from ages 10 to 13), for two weeks in July, I attended Camp Firefly for Children with Diabetes. For two awesome weeks every year, I was just like everyone else! I had diabetes, and I was part of the in-crowd. I was THE MAJORITY, and we ruled.

The girls in my bunk and I tested our blood sugars together, swam together, laughed out loud until we rolled on the floor together (that was possible even in the pre-Internet days), and even made each other cry from time to time. No matter what, we were the FireFly girls and we stuck together. Diabetes camp gave me a swagger in my step and created some of the happiest moments of my childhood!

I remember coming home from camp brimming with confidence! And that confidence stayed with me for a good part of the year. Just when my confidence would start to wane, I'd get a letter or a phone call from one of my Camp Firefly girls, and I was immediately reminded that camp was just around the corner.

The summer before I went into eighth grade was the summer we didn't have the money for me to go to camp. My heart was broken, and my personality changed. I worked as a mother's helper for 20 hours a week instead that summer. Eighth-grade adolescence wasn't kind, and I'd lost the confidence that diabetes camp had given me, not to mention a network of friends and confidants that I still think of to this day.

Bottom line: There's nothing like having a friend (or a gaggle of them) who gets what it's like to have diabetes, especially when you're growing up. Nothing like a friend who understands what it's like to feel low or who can relate to the frustrations of stubborn high blood sugar that won't come down. And there's no place better than a diabetes camp to give your teen some unforgettable summer memories and lifelong friends who understand diabetes.

Kelly Kunik, the creator/author/editrix and siren of the diabetes patient–centric blog Diabetesaliciousness is a passionate diabetes advocate, speaker, writer, and humorist and consults with companies and organizations on the diabetes patient perspective. Kelly grew up in a family where type 1 diabetes roots wrapped tightly around her family tree. Her blog has been featured in numerous publications, including SELF magazine, the LA Times, Healthline.com, and EverdayHealth.com.

CHAPTER SEVEN

Diabetes and School for Teens

When my daughter was a tiny school child, I was lucky enough to convince her public school to hire a full-time aide to stay with her each year. She didn't need that aide all the time, but one could never know exactly when a child with diabetes might need to check or bolus or to eat or more. Since the aide was full-time, my daughter became a sought-after student by teachers. Who didn't want a second pair of hands in the classroom? In any case, "Mrs. D" made school life easy for Lauren, and pretty much stress free for the school nurse and me. Of course we were both involved in the daily routine, but this setup made her at-school diabetes care so much less stressful.

So, when my daughter hit middle school, sat me down before the school year started, and told me matter-of-factly,

"I'm ready to not have an aide anymore," I was crushed. "Well, Mom," she asked, "When would you have wanted me to keep her around until?"

"I don't know," I replied. "Maybe until a few months after you get back from your honeymoon? Or, after you have kids?" Of course I realize how lucky we were to have this aide and how rare this situation was. But still, I wish my now adult daughter still had her.

All joking aside, it's hard to move toward a place where your teen with diabetes does not have constant supervision. And yet, it must eventually happen. For us, the slow move away from the school nurse and toward independence was a necessary yet painful one. The nurse worried a lot; she truly cared about my daughter. (We were lucky enough to have the same school nurse from kindergarten to graduation. Imagine that!) I feared the worst: left to her own devices, she would never do the right thing. And my daughter just chugged along, shaking her head at us all, going about her busy life as a teen and a student.

In the end, as always, it was about balance. We did not have a perfect experience with it, but we did learn. Hopefully this chapter will help you think about how to enable your teen to thrive in school and at work.

And Mrs. D? You're a great aide. Can I ship you down to Lauren's college?

School. It takes up a majority of our teen's time almost every day. For parents of a teen with diabetes, this represents a large span of time when, in reality, parents have little oversight or "control" over their teen and his or her actions. Parents who had their children grow up with diabetes in the school setting got used to the child interacting almost constantly with the school nurse (if a nurse is present) and/or with the other school personnel. This interaction provides a kind of window for the parents to peek through almost any time they want to know what is going on. High school can bring a change—or at least some pushback—in all that.

So how is a parent to manage diabetes, their teen, and the school day? In the case of the long-diagnosed teen, the high school years are probably a time of moving somewhat away from the constant supervision of the nurse. The first reason is usually logistical: teens have to dash from class to class, sometimes a good distance between each classroom and often back and forth across the school throughout the day. It might be just plain hard to find time to get to the nurse's office even once a day, never mind multiple times.

The second reason can often be that it's time. In a few years, kids will be heading off to college or work or whatever life as an adult brings them. High school is a chance to begin the slow march toward independence, and seeing the nurse less can be a part of that march.

The third reason might be more complicated: your teen feels he or she knows more than the school nurse may know. In most cases you have to admit that's probably true. But the school nurse is a valuable tool, if you have one to call on, to have honed and in place, even if it is just for when your teen needs the nurse in a special situation. (We will talk more about the teen with no medical support at school later in this chapter.)

The Teen's Voice in the School Plan

As teens transition through middle school and into high school, that usually means meeting with and building a relationship with a new school nurse, or the person or people the school puts in charge of your child's daily care. For instance, in Texas, all public schools are mandated to have two non-medical people in school who know about T1D. Teens can find this frustrating. They don't want to have to stop and answer questions that they feel medical folks should know; they'd rather not take time to teach someone the basics that seem so obvious to them. But it's just plain smart to do just that. You can tell your teen that helping the nurse get in the know does not mean that nurse will be running your teen's diabetes all day. Rather, it means that teens will have a support system in place on campus for when they need it. Remind your teen that their extra supplies will need to be stored in the nurse's office, and that he or she will want to use the office to do site changes (if pumping) and to seek help if sick or extra high or extra low.

Even if your nurse has experience with other students with T1D, ask for a meeting to discuss your teen's plan. Remind the nurse, in polite terms, that every single person with diabetes is unique, and that while she may have a plan set up with another student that works like a charm, you'll need to work with her to create one that is for your child and your child alone. Take this time to let her know your teen's level of knowledge, and also what in your experience helps or hinders your teen. Without being accusatory, find a way in

Let Your Teen's Voice Lead

True, you are the parent, and you are responsible for making sure all is in place with the school. But in the teen years, involve your teen in the process. This might mean making allowances you've not considered, but let teens be part of educating the nurse and setting up the in-school plan. They'll feel empowered.

advance to help the nurse to keep from nagging your child. Teens dislike it enough when parents say, "Did you forget to check again?" Hearing the school nurse say it only compounds their annoyance.

The big question, of course, boils down to this: will your teen be required to check with a nurse or another adult in the know at some point during each day? This is a decision that you, your teen, and your medical team should make first and foremost. Sure, you want the nurse/school to feel comfortable and secure, but that's not your first priority. If your teen's medical team agrees the teen is capable of checking on his or her own, that's what you should aim for. And if your teen is absolutely insistent on it, find a way to make that happen.

This could be a good "bargaining chip" with teens. Agree they can check on their own, and then set up minimum requirements. For instance, you could say that you need them to check at lunchtime and just before sports practice (or drama club or history study group or whatever else comes after school). In your mind, be aware that there are going to be times when they forget or just blow it off. Consider a "three strikes and you're out" policy. If they forget to check at, say, lunchtime, three times in a month, they'll need to go back to the nurse's office for that lunch check for the following month. Put this in writing between you and your child, not you and the nurse. And if your child does wind up having to go to the nurse for that check for a month, simply tell the nurse you'll be sending the teen in for a few weeks just for your own personal reasons. Put this in writing with your teen, like a contract. And if they have another idea for a plan, listen to it. They might just come up with something better.

For newly diagnosed teens in a school with a nurse in place, daily stops at the nurse's office are probably going to be a must, at least for a period of time. Talk to your teen's medical team, and let your teen share with them the logistics of a typical day. Is he or she worried about being able to make it to the nurse and still have time for lunch each day? Is your teen uncomfortable having to go there constantly? Let them know that in time, most teens can handle things without daily nurse visits, and this hopefully can just be for a period of time. And when you communicate the plan with the nurse, as said before, include your teen. Help teens build an open and confident relationship with those in place to support them.

When There's No School Nurse

More and more often, due to budget cuts and other reasons, teens with diabetes head to school each day without a nurse on duty to assist them. So what if your school has no nurse? If the school will agree, it's a good idea to have some kind of adult in place who can be a sounding board, helper, and assistant to teens when they need it. This will involve training. Some schools agree to have a guidance counselor or lead aide take on that duty. You'll want someone with whom your teen is comfortable and to whom he or she is willing to go when needed.

You'll also need a secure place for your teen to store supplies such as insulin, meter backups, and pump supplies if there is no nurse's office. Refrigeration is needed, but chances are your teen is not the only student in the school who needs medication stored. Find out the current plan and discuss your needs with the principal.

If there is no nurse in place, you'll also need to come up with a way for your teen to communicate with you regularly, at least at the start. Texting, calling, whatever works: you will need them to be sharing as you both learn to manage this during the school day.

The 504 Plan and Older Students

For public school students in the United States, the 504 Plan is a staple for doing well with type 1 diabetes onboard. The 504 is basically a set of rules and rights for your child with diabetes in the school building. It is your job as a parent to draft your child's 504 and work with the school to make sure it is adhered to. (For other countries and private schools, you'll need to discuss a set up with your principal as they are not covered under the 504 laws).

Typical 504s include freedom to eat anywhere in school, to drink water or visit the restroom, to have access to diabetes supplies, and to be allowed to go to the nurse any time it is needed. More expanded 504s include permission to retake tests if a high or low blood sugar inhibits the student's ability during the test, waiver of punishments for excessive absences and tardiness when they are the result of diabetes issues, and sometimes, even, a tutor to help a student who might miss a large amount of time because of diabetes-related sickness. 504 plans can also include permission to use a cell phone for calling or texting about blood sugar levels. Teens need to understand that if they do have this right, it will be taken away in an instant if they abuse it. Understanding their 504 is an important growing step for teens.

A 504 is teens' protection, so that they are treated in a way that is fair while they are in school. But here's the rub: the last thing most teens want to do is "wave the 504 flag." In fact, far from abusing the 504 for special treatment, most teens don't call on it enough. Sometimes this is because the teen does not want to discuss diabetes. But a more common reason might actually be a good one: teens want to move toward a place where they no longer ask for special consideration.

While it is fair and right for teens to use a 504 in high school, teens have a point when they say they eventually will have to work things out in the "real world." For the most part, there are no

"504s" in the work force or even in college, although some colleges now do have a version of a 504 for students with disabilities. If you can, help teens to see that in these years, with standardized testing and other things that impact their future, and since they are still children, it's best to use the 504.

One thing you may want to do is ask teens what they'd like included in their 504. And remind them, if they ask that something not be included, it's better to have too much in there than not enough. But they may have thoughts and ideas about their school day that you don't. And including them is a nice step toward independence and those days down the road when they must advocate for themselves.

Insulin, Needles, Hallways, and Desks, Oh My!

What about carrying diabetes supplies around school? Pumps have changed the rules on self-administering insulin (because really, you cannot go to the nurse every minute the pump sends some basal into your body, and pushing buttons to take your insulin at meal times and when high is a simple task). But what about checking blood sugars and taking shots?

Most school systems today allow students to carry their own supplies as long as they have medical clearance to do so from their medical team, and as long as they have a 504 plan in place saying they can. But at this point in their lives, you need to let teens understand that with this right comes responsibility, and like all rights in life, one must honor the responsibility to maintain the right. Some rules that teens need to abide by when carrying their own diabetes supplies include:

- Dispose of medical waste properly. It is usually best to keep any sharps in their diabetes bag and throw it out at home. They can never, ever, leave a used needle or lancet anywhere in school—including the trash. All school nurse offices should have sharps containers if they ever want to get rid of one in school.
- Do not share. Teen friends love to ask if they can check their blood sugar with the diabetes meter. This can never, ever be done in school or on school property.
- Lock supplies up when they are not in the teen's possession. If, say, a teen is in gym class, medical supplies should always be under lock and key. If it is a problem for the teen to do that, the teen should ask a teacher or coach for help.

Your teen's 504 plan should include permission to carry their medical supplies, along with the right to visit the restroom, drink water, and eat anywhere as needed, as well as possibly use a cell phone to text numbers or questions. With that, too, comes responsibility: your teen cannot abuse these rights. You need to let teens know if they use a cell for things other than is allowed in their 504, they may lose the right to use it at all, which might mean them having to go back to visiting the nurse's office more frequently. Also remind them to be conscientious: if they have to eat in class because of a low, don't leave crumbs or wrappers behind. And don't lord their right to eat in class over other kids. Only use it when needed.

When Only the Nurse's Office Will Do

Of course, there are still going to be times when teens simply must visit the nurse or go to a private place where their medical supplies are stored if a nurse is not in place. And while these are up to you, your teen, and your medical team to decide on, some are commonly shared. For instance, it is best if a teen requiring a change of a pump site uses the nurse's office or a private, set location. It's cleaner, it's quieter, and it provides total privacy. Also, backup pump supplies are stored more easily there than in a backpack or in a purse. While you will still want your teen to have a pump site on hand, have him or her use the nurse's office or a secure supply area and the supplies there if a site change is warranted.

A teen that is particularly high may need to visit the nurse or a private, secure spot to check ketones. While in a perfect world a ketone meter would be available there (because you have it stored there), at the very least if insurance does not allow an extra ketone meter, have ketone urine strips on hand. You will need to come to an agreement with your teen on when ketones must be checked (over a certain blood sugar number, when high two times in a row, or other criteria as decided by your teen's medical team).

> **Buddy System!**
>
> Remember, teens with diabetes need a buddy to walk them to the nurse if they are low or feeling ill from a high. A person with diabetes should not go off alone when in this condition. Write this into a teen's 504 and remind him or her to use it. The buddy system is not just for little kids.

A teen who is low more than once may want to spend some time with the nurse or in a quiet place with adult supervision, at the very least to rest for a bit.

While shots may be taken anywhere (as long as the teen adheres to the rules and has a 504 allowing this), sometimes a teen may want to go to the nurse to take a shot. If this is the case with your teen, work with your nurse to make it seamless and quick. Teens with diabetes don't always want to talk about their entire diabetes day every time they walk in the nurse's room. If it is something routine, encourage your school nurse to give your teen the needed space and some privacy.

Sometimes teens slip in their daily care, too (as discussed in chapter 11). In this case, parents may want to require a teen to check and take insulin in the nurse's office at least one time a day for a period of time. Remember: your nurse can help as another set of eyes when a teen needs that backup.

The "Big" Tests and Diabetes

SATs. ACTs. State exams. Finals. AP tests. Tests for technical programs instead of college. The teen years, particularly the junior and senior years of high school, are full of major exams—ones that take a long time, bring stress, and, yes, matter in their outcome. Planning ahead for these—and learning how your teen does with other kinds of testing with diabetes onboard—is key to success here.

First of all, your teen does have rights when it comes to the big tests such as SATs, ACTs, APs, and the like. It is your duty to contact the board that administers the tests and get the information you need to put any special allowances in place for your teen (such as being able to access food and drink and a glucose meter during the test). It is important to note here that even if

> **Earlier Is Better**
>
> It's a good idea to think way ahead on this one. Contact your school guidance counselor well before exams are coming up and ask for input and past experience the school has had helping students who need accommodations. Better to know the steps ahead of time and be ready.

you have provisions for testing in your teen's 504, you still should contact the testing board and confirm the arrangements. They may ask to check that you do have a 504 on file in some cases. Each testing board has its own web site. You'll get it when your child registers. Simply log on, search for "accommodations," and follow it from there.

That said, many teens opt not to use accommodations (once again wanting to just be "normal"). In most of these test cases, such as the SATs, any child with an accommodation is assigned a special number. When they check in on test day, they will be placed in a separate room from others taking the test (but along with any other student who might have the same accommodation). Some teens like this: a quieter room without anyone else around can help with focus. Others don't. You'll have to discuss this with your teen and see what they'd like to do. They just need to remember that without the accommodations, should they go low or high or need something, they'll have to walk out of the test and negate it, meaning they'll have to take it again (and that costs money, too).

Prepping for the test is the same as for kids without diabetes. You'll want your child to eat a well-rounded breakfast a good half hour or more before the test begins. You should know from experience what blood glucose number truly hinders your teen's ability to focus on a test. But remember: it does not have to be "perfect." Talk to your medical team about what blood sugar they would say means "don't take the test." If your teen is a bit high before the test, consider just letting her or him take it and see what happens. The teen may just do fine.

Blood Sugar Readings and Success at School

There is no way around it: blood sugars close to a reasonable target range do affect how a teen performs, academically and otherwise. This is almost a cruel joke: take young people and place them in the years that perhaps matter most to their academic success (working toward college; wanting to earn their way to the next steps in their lives). Then toss in hormones that mess with blood sugars, moods that mess with a teen's willingness to pay close attention, and a dollop of burnout, and you've got quite a stew of angst there.

How to make it work? First, teens probably already understand that erratic blood sugars affect their performance. Particularly if they've been at this for a while, they've experienced what it's like to lose focus or just be unable to perform at top ability when blood sugars are high or low. But it's okay to remind them. You may want to ask your child's CDE to discuss blood glucose target ranges for testing. Remember here: they may not be what you as a parent would think they need to be. But let your teen learn from their medical team. In other words, there may be a wider range that could be fine while testing. Be open to that possibility.

Of course, theoretically, it's a good idea for your teen to pull out the meter and do a check before any test. Are teens going to do that every time? Probably not. Encourage them to. Let them know that if a pop quiz comes along, you don't necessarily expect them to stop and check. But for something with more weight, such as a midterm, final, or other big exam, if they would be willing to check, it might help them.

So what if they don't check and begin to feel low or unable to focus? You should have in a teen's 504 that he or she can stop a test at any time to check and treat. If teens do this and find they are high or low, or at some point know that their diabetes is affecting the possible outcome, they should stop and let a teacher know.

And again the problem is usually this: teens just don't like waving the 504 flag. While most 504s are written to allow teens to retake a test if afterward they discover they were too high or too low, many teens don't even want to do that, even with teachers begging them to do so.

In the end, all you as a parent can do is have a good plan in place, educate your teen about it, and then let teens decide. After all, if they feel they'd rather sink or swim with diabetes onboard, they really are just moving toward the place in their life when they will, for the most part, have to do just that. It can be frustrating for a parent if a teen does not want to retake a test that may have been affected by diabetes, but in the end, it's a learning experience either way. For instance, the teen that refuses accommodations for the SAT and then tanks because of, say, high blood sugar, usually works hard the next test time to be in a range that might not have an effect. And while we all want our kids to rock every test, if they learn a lesson, the test was a success.

Sports, Activities, and Long Days Away from Home

It is entirely possible that your teen heads out the door at 6:30 a.m. and does not return until 7 p.m. With sports, clubs, drama, jobs, and more, teens are busy—and away from watchful parents—often 50 percent of the day or longer. So how do you keep them safe and healthy at school after the school nurse has checked out for the day? Much of this of is going to fall on your teen and you (or another adult).

Sports and programs such as drama, student government, art clubs, and study groups happen on school grounds. Most schools have an athletic trainer on site and in place while sports are going on. This is the person you should befriend and educate about your child. (Even if the child is in, say, drama and not sports, this person can help you.) In a perfect world, they'd be willing to be trained in how to use a glucagon, and even let you keep one stored in their medical case.

What about coaches and club advisors? Some parents have success in asking those people to be trained in glucagon, but others do not. At the very least, adults overseeing your teen's activities after school should be required by the 504 plan to learn and know anything the teachers who supervise them during the school day know. That means they should understand your child's rights and needs; that sometimes the teen may need to stop practice and check blood sugars and eat, but that they will probably be fine in a short time. Similar to the school day, your child should not be punished when this happens.

But the teen who takes on extra programs needs to accept some responsibility, too. Any teen who joins a sports team or a club realizes this in general: joining and dedicating themselves means they'll have to work to find other times to study and do homework and keep their grades up. Most, if not all, schools require a minimum grade point average to take part in such things. They'll also commit to keeping their uniforms clean and bringing it when they need it, to making practices regularly, and to being a positive example of the team in the community.

So if you talk over some diabetes responsibilities with them, it probably won't be the first time they've agreed to go an extra mile to be part of the programs they choose. What do they need to do? It's perfectly reasonable that you expect them to check their blood sugars at the end of the school day and before they begin their activity or sport. The school day is a long one, and they'll want to be sure to know where they are at numbers-wise before starting the next part of their day.

Of course they also need to be responsible and have with them anything they might need—fast-acting carbs, strips for the meter, the meter itself, insulin, and a backup pump site change if they are pumping. Most parents of teens do not mind checking their teen's bag to make sure this stuff is stocked up. After all, we are all forgetful, and teens have so much going on with classes, games, events, and more. It's not overbearing to make sure they have what they need on hand at all times.

When a game or even a practice stretches into the early evening, you'll want your teen to check again. Your best bet is discussing a plan ahead of time and asking teens what they feel would work. And of course, when food is involved, you'll want them to remember to take their insulin. Carb-counting programs on their smartphone can help them know what they are eating. As is always the case, don't expect them to be perfect at all times. The best thing you can hope for is a reasonable effort backed by honesty. If you can encourage your teen to be honest ("We had pizza on the way home from the show and I did not check or bolus. Now I'm high."), your parental response should not be "You can never go again now!" Rather, take a breath and say, "Okay, check now and let's get that corrected. Thanks for giving me a heads-up." Easier said than done, but the teen who is supported and not judged is going to be honest more often.

The school day is, perhaps, the largest part of your teen's life for ten months of the year. Finding a way to keep teens on track during those hours is a lesson in itself. And since school is practice for the working world, you'll be helping your teen learn to live out there in the big world.

> **Checking in with You?**
>
> Of course you want to ask teens to text, e-mail, or call with blood sugar readings during the day. But consider not doing so. You can look at their meter in the evening, and if they need advice, they can call you. Let them feel independent here.

CHAPTER EIGHT

Diabetes, the Teen, and Making a Social Life Work

My daughter with diabetes was born a social animal. She had a posse of friends five rows deep and a social calendar that spread out over months, it seemed, from the time she was born. I realized early on in our life with diabetes that balancing all that with safe, decent diabetes care was going to be a challenge.

If I had left it up to her, it probably would not have been a big deal: she's always been one to just roll with the social scene and live life by the moment. But I'm her mom and protector. My first thought was to just keep her at home. She could have playgroups over here, I thought. She can host all the high school parties here, too. We'll add on. Maybe even the school's extracurricular events could happen right here in *my own living room, where I knew she was safe and within a few feet of me.*

Of course, this was just silly fantasy. The reality is that we have to let our kids go, and the social part of their lives is possibly the most important thing on their minds. Consider this: a study done on teens with dangerous food allergies and their parents told the tale of what goes on in the minds of both. When asked what was the most important goal in their teen lives with food allergies onboard, a vast majority of teens said building a great, exciting, and fulfilling social life without the allergies getting in the way of that. The parents? Asked their number one goal for their teens at this time, a vast majority responded with "keeping them alive."

In other words, while parents were worried about allergies killing their kids, the kids were worried about it killing their social lives. Talk about not working in tandem.

The same could be said for living with diabetes. We parents think first of our child's safety, and well we should. We are their defensive line in this world, tackling problems as they come along. How are we to do that if their social lives keep them away from us, crazy busy and on a schedule we cannot possibly always keep up with?

For us, the answer was simple. Well, like most things with diabetes onboard, it was complicatedly simple. I had to let her go. I had to let her live, which meant going to overnights, parties, jobs, events, and places I could not control.

In her teen years I let her sleep over at the homes of friends I had not known before; attend a two-week leadership conference in Washington, D.C., basically on her own (which led her to find the college she wanted to attend and the career she wanted to pursue—worth every moment of worry); stay out all night on prom night; and more. It wasn't easy, but it was right.

Because in the end, we are raising a person to be happy, smart, healthy, and fulfilled. It's not just about the blood sugar value, although there are ways to try to keep that in line, too. This chapter looks at the relationship between diabetes and a teen's larger social life and hopefully gives you the courage (because it does take parental courage) to let your child savor the entire teen experience.

Who ever said great parenting was easy? It's not.

Helping your teen make his or her social life work is one of your most important jobs. Of course, this often means taking leaps of faith that you simply never had to take when your teen was younger. But understanding what different parts of teens' social lives might mean and helping them think ahead to events and situations could make a big difference.

Your teen's endocrinology team can play a major role in this, too. It is their job, as much as it is yours, to help your teen navigate new situations and plan for special events they might want to take part in. Can they have the total spontaneity of a teen without diabetes? Well, no. But it's important for them—and you—to remember that all teens need parental oversight and support, not just teens with diabetes. So while the details may differ from those of others, your teen needs to realize that all caring parents give advice, ask questions, and make sure situations are safe and proper for their teens. It's not just the diabetes that drives you to guide them, in other words.

Overnights and School Trips: How to Say Yes

What is it about kids and sleepovers? Even without diabetes along, they are rife with issues. Kids come home tired and cranky. They eat less than optimally. Often, there's bickering in the middle of it all. Why do kids love them so much? And yet they do. A sleepover is a bonding experience and part of growing up. Yet many parents of teens with diabetes fear letting them go off to sleep over somewhere.

So how do you say yes? First of all, technology makes this all easier. Remember, with cell phones and texting, your teen is never really out of touch with you. It's simple enough to know what is going on and keep tabs if that is what you want.

But first, here are the musts of sleepovers that your teen should agree to in order to be able to go (and consider this: most if not all of these would be musts even if your teen did not have diabetes).

- You must speak with the parent in charge first. Why? Because you need to make sure your child and his or her friends are being honest about what they are doing. (Yes, that's hard to grasp, but it's your job to check in and make sure everything is on the up and up. If your child lied about where he or she was going, they would not be the first to have ever done that.) A phone call a day ahead of time to the parent in charge at the home must happen, even if your teen pitches a fit about it. You can let your teen know this actually has little to do with diabetes—you'd be doing it anyway. It's what cautious parents do.

- The parent in charge must know your child has diabetes. This is non-negotiable. You don't need to go into the details of how to care for a child with diabetes, nor do you need to train the parent in giving shots or treating lows (more on that in a bit). But it is your obligation to let the parent know. If there ever were to be a problem—goodness forbid—it would be grossly unfair for that parent not to have had a heads-up prior to the evening. Your teen may blanch at this. But tell teens it's just simply the polite thing to do. You can give them the option to tell the parents on their own, but you need to confirm that has happened. Remember to tell the parent that your child can eat anything any other child does and does not need the parent to provide "special food." Remember, most people do not know this.

- Your teen must set up with you an agreed-to plan for diabetes care that evening. Don't expect teens to be perfect; just look for them to be safe. You know they'll probably be eating chips and other things that make keeping track difficult. Don't demand they count out chips into a bowl and eat only those. Instead, ask for them to check at certain times and text you. Let them know you can text them back a suggested course of action. Sometimes this is more agreeable to teens, since it means they don't have to talk out loud about what they are dealing with in the middle of all the fun. And make sure they know you don't expect their blood sugars to be perfect that night. After all, life is about savoring it while doing your best.

What if you are a parent who does regular middle-of-the-night checks (some parents do, and some parents do not? How can your teen spend the night where you are not)? A first idea may be simple: skip the night check. Talk to your endo team and ask them if they feel this is a good idea. If they say it is, go for it. There is going to have to be a time your child moves on to not having you there all night. A sleepover close by could be a first experience with that. A second idea is to ask them to set an alarm and do it themselves. You could choose to either have them text or call you at that time or just let you see the meter the next day.

- Your teen must check by an agreed-upon time in the morning and give you a quick call or text. Sleepovers usually mean no sleep all night and then crashing in the morning. Explain to your teen that, silly you, you'll be worried in the morning. Set an alarm on a cell phone and ask the teen to wake up, quickly check, text, and then go back to sleep. Put it on you: say you are such a worrywart that it will just make your morning more relaxing. (And it will.) Laugh about it. Tell them you just need them to do it, period.

Beyond that, it's up to you to let your child prove him- or herself. Let teens know that while you do not expect perfection (there is no such thing as perfection in diabetes anyway), you do expect them to do the bare minimum: check the number of times you've agreed on (or at least most of those times) and be sensible while having fun. As time goes on and they attend more overnights, let them know you will get more relaxed about it (but the rules above will always stand).

What if something goes wrong at a sleepover, such as drinking or sneaking out to walk through town in the middle of the night? First of all, let your teen know if they feel unsafe or do not want to take part in that, they can "use the diabetes card" to get out. This does not mean saying, "I have diabetes. I can't" Rather, it means saying, "I'm having some issues with my blood sugars and I need to call my mom. Sorry guys, I have to go home."

Of course, there is more of a chance your teen is going to want to take part in some sneakiness. Here's the key to that: let teens know they can always be honest with you. If they make a mistake at a party and confess it to you, stay calm and discuss what happened and how things went. It is much better to have honesty, which could mean your teen calls you or admits to an unsafe situation that you can help them learn from. Remind them, too, that they have a permanent "get out of jail free card" with you. If they drink at a party or do something else they should not have, calling you immediately for help means they will not be severely punished. There could be consequences (like deciding they might not be ready for an overnight with a lack of supervision), but they should never fear asking you for help in a critical situation.

> ### Building Trust, One Night at a Time
>
> Sleepovers and other events are a chance for your teen to build trust with you and for you to allow the teen to do so. As teens get older, do let them take the lead on some of these things. Give them a chance (or two or three) to do it right. Show them that trust helps win freedom from your constant oversight.

What about overnights such as all-night prom parties? Again, as always, you want to take diabetes out of the equation and ask yourself: would I let my teen go without diabetes? If the answer is yes, you need to let the teen go. For such events, you can volunteer to be a chaperone. But, if your child does not want you to, step out of the picture. As in the case of the slumber party at a house, you'll need to let the parent in charge know your child has diabetes. Again, they don't need to know details. Here, good friends can be a great tool. As we discussed in chapter 6, longtime friends (and not all kids are lucky enough to have been in one place for a long time or kept such relationships) are often willing to know how to use glucagon, to look out for problems, and even to quietly get your teen to check a few times during such an event. Do enlist their help and trust them to help you keep your teen happy and safe. Friends can be the best tool a family with diabetes can have. That also models for teens what they need to do as they move forward in life. Having friends who understand, are educated, and are willing to help is what adults with diabetes do.

School Trips

Many high schools—and even middle schools—hold overnight trips to everything from camps for nature study to big cities such as Washington, D.C., New York City, Chicago, Seattle, and other historical and educational spots. And while some schools do send school nurses on the trips, others do not.

So what are you to do? Make a plan, talk it out, and then let them go. These school trips can actually be great practice for what is looming down the road … college. There, we said it. College is looming down the road, and you need to help your teen with diabetes prepare for that next step.

You first need to find out what kind of medical support accommodations your school makes for such trips. If there is a nurse going along, your decision was just made easier. You will need to have a meeting with the nurse to discuss your child's diabetes plan during the trip. And you may have to make some compromises. For instance, if you are a parent who checks your child in the middle of the night, you may need to find a way to skip that check or help your child to do it on his or her own. Cell phone alarms can be set if you want your child to do the check. You could even set an alarm for the same time and be awake for it while at home. Or, you could consider letting your teen try sleeping without the middle-of-the-night check. It's a good idea with a trip like this to discuss it ahead of time with your CDE or another member of the medical team. Since they know your child and your family, they can help you come up with a plan (and they've seen this before and have good input to give).

What if there is no nurse and your child does not want you to be a chaperone? A middle school student may be too young to be on their own with diabetes. It's an individual decision that needs to be made by you, the medical team, and your child. If you can take the time and your child does not mind you chaperoning, tell her or him that you'll leave some space and just be there to help, and not to nag or constantly be by the child's side. But teens in high school may very well be ready for their first adventure with diabetes along and no medical support right there.

If you do decide this, the adult in charge will need to be briefed on the details. And teens will need to (even if it annoys them to the nth degree) sit down and talk out a plan for the trip with you. It's okay to expect them to check in: texting makes it easier. Even if they end up busy at a time when you wanted them to call, a quick text can let you know that.

Food will be a challenge on the trip. While you can probably get a schedule of where they'll be eating and when, you won't be able to control what your child chooses. Be sure your child has a good carb-counting app on a cell phone (you know teens will never forget their phone anywhere, whereas they might easily forget a small book with carb counts). If you can, make a list of their favorites that you see them order often when out, and compile that list ahead of time on the app. And remind teens to count their carbs as best they can.

You may also want to talk to their medical team about a higher blood sugar range during the trip. Lows tend to be the biggest worry parents have. If your team agrees your child could run at a higher range for the time gone, go along with it. Diabetes is a marathon, not a sprint. And it's okay to see higher numbers from time to time if it means it's helping them move toward freedom and responsibility.

At the end of it all, praise teens once they are home. Don't expect their numbers to be perfect and don't freak out if they missed a check here and there. In fact, simply praise them for doing it, no matter how it looks on paper. What parents need to realize is that as much as teens may beg to get freedom, it's challenging and frightening for them, too. Their first big trip away from home is a reason to celebrate and congratulate. Be sure to do just that. Because in the end, our goal is to set our kids free. A trip like this could be just the thing to start those wings sprouting.

> **The Diabetes Parent "Network"**
>
> There are parents of kids with diabetes in every city. Our world of connectedness means we either know them or know someone who knows them. Consider finding a "diabetes parent" nearby where your child will be going and ask that person to be on call in case your child needs something. Offer to return the favor or pay it forward when a teen is near your neck of the woods.

Food and the Teen's Social Life

Remember when you planned out every meal, even when you went out to eat? Now your teen is dashing around, grabbing pizza or other fast food with friends, stopping in the coffee shop for a snack, and gobbling down goodies friends bring to the beach or the lake or the game to share. What's a parent to do? First off, try to set up your teen with the best tools for success. Apps with carb counts are free and readily available, and most teens have smartphones now. Help your teen download an app and then encourage its use.

Of course, even with an app and the carb amounts of every food at their fingertips, covering all foods precisely would mean teens have to pay careful attention to what is eaten (how many pizza slices was that?), which is hard to achieve. So what's a teen to do? Some parents adopt the "okay if a bit high now, we can correct later" plan. If your teen is heading out, say, to the beach with friends, encourage counting and planning, but let teens know that once they are home, you can always do a correction if they run high. In the end, it is better to come back a bit high than risk a low by over-bolusing for foods they end up not eating.

That said, not covering at all for foods can be a big reason for elevated A1Cs. It's easy for a teen to forget. After all, you've made diabetes simply a "part of their lives," and it's good that they don't overstress about it. But if they can find a way to remember to work at covering a meal or snack, they are going to feel better and fare better.

And what about the "grazing" most teens like to do with foods—snacking and picking and the like? This can even happen at home, while doing homework or just watching television. It's hard to say they cannot graze, because (thanks to the mysterious teen mind) this usually only makes them want to graze more. At home is a good place to "practice." Encourage teens to think about what they might want to eat that afternoon and then see if they can feel like they are grazing while sticking to a planned carb count. It's probably not going to work perfectly, but if they can get used to the idea of at least a starting bolus of insulin for grazing, that might help form good habits when away from you.

You have probably realized over the years that your teen has certain "red-light foods" that spike their blood sugar more than most others. Rather than tell your child never to have them, just educate teens that those foods require more insulin than others. Remind them that every time they eat, say, Chinese food, they usually come in high later. Just knowing that will help them think more about their choices and their decisions regarding those choices—at least in time.

Are there foods you should say "never" to? Possibly. Some diabetes doctors warn against sugary drinks with no added benefits, such as regular soda or slushies, which can cause fast spikes in blood sugars. (Of course when a teen is low, those drinks can be a good choice, only confusing a teen even more.) You may want to have some "suggestions" for your teen to consider. And make them aware that many of the coffee drinks teens now love have way, way more carbs than they even realize. Educate them on what those drinks have in them, and encourage them to try different choices. Don't say never; just say, "Try to limit those to every great once and a while." And model for them by ordering

> **Beware the "Rage Bolus"**
>
> Many teens choose to just give themselves a giant bolus of insulin and then eat what they want. This is not a good choice and should be avoided. Remind them it is better to correct a high two hours later than suffer a low sooner.

the "skinny" choice yourself at the coffee house.

In the end, we all want our teens to grow up with healthy eating habits, coupled with a healthy relationship with food. It's not that much different with diabetes onboard. Your teen will learn, in time, that some foods make them high and are (temporarily) worth it; others do not. Just getting them to pay attention to that goes a long way.

Dating—It's Going to Happen

Your son or daughter with diabetes is going to start dating. The best advice is simple: go on every single date with them, forever and ever.

Okay, not really. And as tempting at that may be, it's best for teens to enter the dating world on their own two feet. But not without some thought.

The first big question parents have about dating is simple: how soon does the person the child is dating need to know about the diabetes? In most cases, dates come from within a current social circle, so most are already aware a teen has diabetes. That said, if the date does not know, in this case it is *completely up to your teen to tell or not tell*. Of course you hope the teen will tell the date, and you will share that hope. Remind your teen that the sooner it's out in the open, the less of a big deal it is. (Think of it this way: if a teen holds off on telling a boyfriend or girlfriend about it, said friend may think "Gosh, it must be bad if they waited so long to tell me.")

And what about teens doing all they have to do while on a date? Sometimes when starting a romantic relationship, teens may not want to show all their needs. Things they have done with barely a thought in the past—such as checking blood glucose at the table, wearing a pump where it can be seen, or even taking a shot—may become something that they feel strange about. In a perfect world, your teen will realize that diabetes care is simply what they have to do, and just go ahead and do it all in front of their date. But teens seldom think in "perfect world" terms.

You may want to ask your teen if they are checking or taking shots in front of their new boyfriend or girlfriend. If they say no, rather than react, simply ask them how they handle it. By stepping into another room? By checking less? By skipping shots or pump boluses? Encourage them to be honest with you. Then suggest they find a way to try to do it in front of the date. Remind them that most of their friends find their diabetes care to be "no big deal," so this new special friend will probably be the same.

What about Sex?

Again, just go with your teen on every single date forever and this will not be a worry. If only.

Teen girls with diabetes need to think particularly carefully about sex. While it is absolutely doable for a woman with T1D to have a baby in today's world, it is still something that needs to be planned out, thought of, and worked out well before conception. In fact, unplanned pregnancies in women with T1D have a higher chance of producing babies with birth defects. Pure and simple, your daughter needs to know this. And really, you need to develop an open and frank discussion about sex with her that's ongoing. While abstinence is always the best choice, better that she be honest with you and get the help she needs before she has sex.

What about contraception? While your daughter is a minor this is an issue that you can have some say in. But it's a good idea to let a teen talk to her pediatrician and/or endocrine team about

It just never seemed like a big deal.

Or at least it never seemed like something I was supposed to hide.

It has always been a part of my life, for as long as I can remember. Every birthday party, every holiday, and every day at school was one with diabetes. That doesn't mean it was an intrusive, offending attendant, but it was there nonetheless. That is how diabetes has affected my life since I was a little kid—it's just a part of what's going on. Testing blood sugars, taking insulin, and managing all these numbers. It was as much a part of my childhood as playing in the yard and riding my bike.

For me, life has always included diabetes. Which means that the lives of those who love me include diabetes, too.

Some people with diabetes keep that information to themselves, disclosing at discreet intervals and building up to a comfortable moment of "telling." Others wear their diabetes diagnosis on their sleeves and make it part of their introductions. It can be a clumsy conversation, or it can be handled with confidence, but being close with people means they know what your life involves. For me, diabetes is something that needs to be disclosed almost immediately. Love me, love my diabetes.

But when it came to dating, I didn't want it to be a "love my diabetes" *focus*. It's not about diabetes. It's not like "Kerri" and "diabetes" have to be separate entities, just like "writer" and "uncoordinated" and "messy hairdo in the morning" and "hot-tempered" remain parts of my whole. I'm one big mess, and I wanted my romantic partners to be into all of me, including the diabetes part.

Mostly, during my dating years, I wanted diabetes to be just this *thing*, this small thing that was such a wee part of the adjective list someone who loved me would use to describe me. I didn't want to ever be defined by my broken pancreas; I wanted to be seen as so many other things first. Diabetes was, and is, a big part of my life, but it's not the core of who I am. And it won't ever be.

When it comes to my husband, I sometimes take his view on diabetes for granted. I don't tell him how much he means to me as often as I should. He is a wonderful partner. There's all the regular relationship stuff—he pumps the gas for my car so I don't have to stand in the cold, he takes out the garbage, he laughs at my stupid jokes, he reads my written messes and helps me make sense of them—but our relationship has an extra, special component that others don't.

He is the significant other of a person with diabetes.

I don't know what it's like to fill that role. I am the diabetic, so I only know things from my perspective. But he makes it look so easy. A 3 a.m. low blood sugar that has me in tears? He knows how to quickly give me juice and wipe the sweat from my forehead. Weeks of working out with no visible results? He knows what words will soothe me: "You are healing from the inside out." Those moments when I feel like I'm crumbling emotionally? His hugs seem to put my pieces back together again.

And it's not just the serious stuff. We aren't always talking about complications and fears. He makes this diabetes stuff feel so normal. He makes me feel like everyone is wearing multiple devices attached to their body when they climb into bed. Disconnecting a pump before sex? Who doesn't do that? Cookies on the bedside table? Not kinky—proactive!

Chris celebrates the victories with me. When my wedding dress was perfectly fitted with a pocket to conceal my pump, he knew that was an important moment. When the Dexcom shows a nice, nine-hour flatline, we do a dance. And when my A1C remained tightly controlled and steady throughout my pregnancy with our daughter, we celebrated our healthy baby with huge smiles (and a severe lack of sleep).

Even though his pancreas works properly, he lives with diabetes, too; just as every loving caregiver of a patient with diabetes lives with diabetes. They don't feel the highs and lows as acutely as we do, but they have their own individual variations on these moments that are just as poignant and just as evocative. Chris understands what this disease means and how it can unfold, but he's as committed to my health and to my life as I am.

And that, to me, is what love with diabetes is all about.

Kerri Sparling has been living with T1D for over 26 years. She believes: "Diabetes doesn't define me, but it helps explain me." Kerri is the creator of www.SixUntilMe.com, started in May 2005. She has contributed to many health-related publications and is a passionate advocate for diabetes awareness. Focusing on the psychosocial side of diabetes and how peer-to-peer connections can impact diabetes management, Kerri presents regularly at conferences and currently works full-time as a writer and consultant.

it without you in the room. If she does need it, better that she ask and get it than not. Do run any decision by your teen's endo team so they can be sure the choice of contraception works well with insulin (and most do).

Expect your son or daughter's endocrine team to begin discussions about sex at a young age. It is their job, too, to make sure the teens are thinking the right way and taking precautions. This is a big reason why, as children near the teenage years, many practitioners begin having part of the appointments without the parent in the room. It's better teens talk to someone than no one. If they are too shy or scared to speak of things with you, be glad there is someone with whom they can speak about it.

Boys, too, need to think about sex. First of all, sexually transmitted diseases can be tougher to deal with when you have diabetes onboard.

And in a simpler way: sex expends energy. You don't want your child to go low and then hop behind the wheel of a car because he doesn't realize that. Talk to teens about it, or have someone talk to them about it.

Boys can also get hung up on erectile dysfunction. It seems that every sporting event on television is now peppered with commercials about drugs for men who suffer from it, and most of them mention diabetes as a cause. It is important that you let your son know that this is most likely *not* going to be their fate. Explain that the commercial is for older men, most of whom do not have diabetes, and many of whom if they do have diabetes had it before the advent of meters and better insulins and pumps. Like many complications, ED could be a thing of the past once your son grows up. He might need to be told that.

In the end, the message your teens with diabetes need to get is the same at its core as all teens: They are not ready for sex. There will be a time. There will be a person. If they can just wait, they'll see the beauty in that one day.

Overseeing without Hovering

So how is a parent to know all is going well in a teen's social life when diabetes is a concern? Just as with a child without diabetes, it is no longer your time to step in and make everything fair on the playground. As a teen, your child must begin to take the steering wheel in his or her social situations and relationships. However, there are ways to help without hovering.

First, share and communicate. It sounds so simple, but with teens who often like to stomp up the stairs, slam the door, and turn on the music, it is not always that easy. Be sure to have time when you are together. Car rides. A lunch or dinner once a week (even if you have to drag the teen there screaming). A walk around the block (ditto even if the teen starts screaming).

Share stories of your life with your teen. See if you can get the teen to share. And do not make it all about diabetes. Make it about life, because you are raising an entire child, not just a child with a disease.

Of course, cell phones do offer us more of a chance to know what is going on. And while you can use that to your advantage, be sure to remember to give your teen some space, too. If you are there to support them and listen, if you don't push too hard, and if you don't invade what really should be teens' time without you, you may just find they're willing to share.

At least a little bit.

CHAPTER NINE

The Big "D"–Driving and Diabetes

I can remember the first day my older daughter, the one without diabetes, pulled out of the house behind the wheel of a car, her little sister in the passenger seat and not a single adult in the car. I was terrified. And my husband, well, he quickly jumped in his car and followed them all over town, two or three cars behind, carefully watching every turn and signal.

Eventually, we got used to it, and our daughter driving off in the car was no different (well, almost no different) from when she used to head out on her bicycle. So when our second daughter earned her license, one would think we'd be more at ease.

But we weren't. Because our second daughter would be

driving with diabetes along. But while we were scared, worried, and stressed, our goal was (as it always has been) to try to help her do everything a child without diabetes would do. We would not hold her back from driving because of our fear.

We found that setting rules on paper and then sticking to them helped. We also affirmed that driving is a privilege, not a right, and took away her privilege when she did not follow those agreed-upon rules.

Today, she's a smart, careful driver. Although I think if my husband had it his way, he'd be right there all the time, two or three cars behind, monitoring every move. Kind of a metaphor for life, eh?

It's one of the life events that teens approach with the most excitement, but parents of teens with diabetes approach with the most trepidation: winning the privilege of driving a car.

It's scary enough to think of any teen behind the wheel of a giant hunk of steel; adding diabetes to the equation, as always, magnifies that fear. Learning to drive and then obeying the rules of the road is something all teens must take seriously. Cars can be dangerous when not operated correctly. It is fair to say that driving a car is the first major responsibility and privilege a person can earn in life. But notice we didn't say winning the "right," but rather "privilege." It is important for parents and teens to realize that driving is not a right but a privilege one earns. Even people without diabetes have to prove themselves before driving and can be stripped of that privilege at any time. Parents should think of this time as a chance to get a foothold on some diabetes rules, since most teens truly yearn to get a driver's license. The strong parent sets up rules of the road (in concert with the medical team and the teen) and then insists that they be kept. This is easier said than done (after all, moms and dads do tire of having to drive kids everywhere and look forward to the freedom of having their children drive on their own), but if you can come up with a plan and stick to it, driving can help a teen and their diabetes. Of course, there are rules you make and rules the state makes. All must be considered.

The Law and Driving with Diabetes

Yes, you absolutely can earn a driver's license if you have diabetes. But in many states there are rules and restrictions in place, and they vary from state to state. For instance, in Texas and Minnesota, a person with diabetes must present the Department of Motor Vehicles (DMV) with a physician's note before earning a driver's license. In Massachusetts and Connecticut, you must only answer "yes" or "no" to a question of whether you've ever had an incident that hindered your ability to drive a vehicle. California has the strictest rules of all. There, any medical person who treats a severe low (as in seizure) by law must report that incident to the DMV, *even if that person was not driving at the time.* That law has been tested by many, but at the time of printing, it still stands. Some states ask vague questions that can be answered in many ways. If your state is one of these, you'll want to discuss with your teen how to best answer.

Your first step as a parent is to get online and look up your own state's driving laws when it comes to diabetes. First and foremost, those must be met. It's a good idea to research them early and discuss them with your teen. Print them out, too, since teens tend to not believe it until they see it. Read these over carefully so your teen fully understands the requirements and the law. That way there can be no doubt later on if a teen claims never to have been told the details.

The law comes into play *after* a teen with diabetes earns his or her license, too. If your teen should go low and crash, he or she can be held accountable by the law. Like it or not, your teen needs to understand that driving while low is not that different than driving drunk. Teens' instincts and motions are impaired, and behind the wheel of a car that can spell danger. It is imperative that teens understand that they simply must be super-responsible about their blood sugars when they drive.

> **The Laws in Your State**
>
> For a state-by-state listing of laws pertaining to driving with diabetes, go to *www.diabetes.org/living-with-diabetes/know-your-rights/discrimination/drivers-licenses/drivers-license-laws-by-state.html.* There you will find up-to-date details about every state.

Learning to Drive

Yes, diabetes complicates everything. And because of that, you'll need to have your own "family driver's ed" before your teen even sits behind the wheel of a car. You'll need to go over point by point the laws about driving with diabetes as well as your own personal rules, and then put it all down on paper. So what rules should you personally consider placing on your teen driver with diabetes?

The first rule is simple: teens *must* check their blood sugar just before getting behind the wheel. It's a good idea to set their target range a little higher than it usually is. For instance, if you and your medical team consider anything below 100 to be a treatable low, make it 130 or even 150 when driving. (Again, make this decision with your teen and the medical team.) You'll also need to set a time limit after which they need to check again if driving a long distance.

Make this decision based on their high and low patterns. Kids love to cruise around at night. If your teen with diabetes is the one behind the wheel, that's going to mean more checks.

The second rule is just as simple: they must wear or carry a recognizable medical alert ID. It can be a bracelet, necklace, charm, wallet card; whatever you agree to it being. But any time your teen is behind a wheel, the medical ID must be worn. Some parents now feel that an insulin pump works the same as a medical ID, but it does not. Teens need to wear the ID for their well-being and protection. A bonus to this is that most teens scoff at the idea of wearing or carrying medical alerts. The lure of driving can bring them back to agreeing to do so.

The third rule is all about preparation: Teens need to make sure they have fast-acting glucose in the car and at their reach at any time. While you as a parent can certainly take on the responsibility of making sure there are glucose tablets in all the cars your teen may be driving, it is his or her duty to double check and know where they are before they drive off to wherever they are going. Glucose tabs are a better choice than juice boxes or crackers, since they don't go bad as quickly and are easy to grab and use.

New Fast-Acting Glucose Products Are Out

Glucose tabs are not the only easy choice now. A new product called Glucostix is now on the market. Kind of like the pixie sticks you may have loved as a kid, they are an easy to digest fast-acting choice.

Even if your teen hates them at home, you may want to suggest their use in the car. So, too, teens should always remember to have a meter and strips on hand, as well as insulin.

The fourth rule is about what to do if teens begin to not feel well while driving. Since highs or lows can happen even when you've checked, educate teens on how to react. First, they need to pull over to a safe place the moment they begin to feel the least bit off. Drive them around town and on the highway and show them where safe pull-off areas are and how to access them. And when you do your driving time with them, do "practice drills" from all kinds of different roads. As your teen drives, say, "Okay, you are feeling low right now. Show me how you'll react." Help teens learn by doing and they'll be better prepared if that should happen.

They need to know that once they pull over to a safe place, they should check blood sugar and then take any action they deem appropriate. And then they should wait 15 minutes and check again, even if they are going to be late to work or the game or school or a date. It's not a bad idea if they call you to check in, too, just so you know what's going on and can help them if needed.

You'll need to remind your teen of that old saying "when in doubt, treat." Behind the wheel more than almost anywhere else, this is the case. If they feel they are going low, and although a check does not indicate it and they have remaining doubts, tell them to grab the glucose supply and go for it. Any high can be corrected once the car is parked and they are safe at their destination.

Of course these are just diabetes-related rules. The many others that they need to learn (speeding, alcohol and driving, wearing a seatbelt, no texting or cell phones, and more) are all part of teaching any child to drive. But it's not a bad idea to include these in your educating as you go along as well.

It's in the Contract

So how do you make all this happen? With a driving contract. You'll find a sample at the end of this chapter. Feel free to use it as a starting point and draft your own.

It's a great idea to involve your teen in the creation and adoption of the contract. You can encourage teens to do some research to come up with some ideas about what they should be expected to do and what kind of results may come if they break any of the contract items. This kind of buy-in helps a teen learn exactly why you are doing something that their friends' parents might not be doing (although, don't you think every teen could benefit from a family driving contract? Just another way life with diabetes sometimes forces us to do even better than most for our children.). It also can help the teen accept the contract as a mutual decision and not something being dictated.

However, the contract is not optional, nor are the items related to diabetes safety while driving. If your teen refuses to accept those mentioned above, he or she is not ready to drive. Period. Because like it or not, these teens have an added layer of responsibility while behind the wheel. And if they balk at the idea, remind them of this: Every single driver in the United States signs a "contract" to drive once the driving test is passed. Theirs just has an addendum. So make it happen, print it out, and have both of you sign it. Keep it on hand. Treat it as real, because it is.

Then, live by the contract. If your teen breaks a rule, follow through. This can be difficult for parents, who have been shuttling their child around for their entire lives and finally get a break. But stick with it you must. Often, it takes only one time losing the right for a teen to get the message. And their safety is worth any inconvenience that might come your way as a parent.

At Required Driver's Ed

And what about driver's education and driver training time? Most states require this for anyone under 18 applying for a driver's license. While it may complicate things, it is your child's responsibility to let their driver's ed teacher know that he or she has type

1 diabetes. Notice we said your teen's responsibility and not yours. If a teen is too shy or immature to discuss diabetes with a driver's education teacher, he or she probably is not ready to learn to drive and apply for a driver's license.

Teens should let the driver's ed teacher know that their parents and medical team have worked with them on the rules of the road with diabetes, and that they will be following them. They should show the teacher how they check before they drive, and how they have glucose on hand in case they need it. From there, if the instructor has more questions, your teen can refer the instructor to you. But in the end, it will be good practice for your teen to do the education here. After all, as a licensed driver, he or she may have to do just that in other situations in the future.

Other than that, the driving instructor should focus on what he or she would be teaching any teen. It is the instructor's job to teach your teen all the other rules of the road and the details of operating a vehicle, but not to teach them how to drive with diabetes along.

When to Say No

That all sounds so simple, but with teens and diabetes, saying and doing are often two separate things. However, with driving, parents really do hold the ultimate control. Make sure your teen knows this is a one-strike-and-you're-out situation. If teens drive the car without checking, they won't be driving for a while. Period. Remember, your action is for the safety of not only your teen but any passengers and the general public.

This can sound daunting, but parents should see this as a chance to reach their teens. Teens are very in-the-moment. No articles about complications or lectures about long-term results of poor control are going to get through to many of them. But the privilege to drive a car? Now that resonates. Use that power for good.

Driving is a normal part of growing up. With some extra layers and an airtight contract, you and your teen can not only survive it but make it work even better than a family teaching a teen without diabetes the rules of driving. Like so many other instances, your teen can be a role model. Remember to tell them that, and to praise them as they do well with their driving.

DRIVING CONTRACT

I, _____ , on this day do agree to the stipulations stated before rendering me the privilege of driving my parents' cars. If, at any time, I violate the said agreement, the driving privilege will be forfeited to the extent and degree of the violation.

1) The use of cellular phones in cars are for your safety and, to let us know of your whereabouts—not for conversation. I will make outgoing calls only for issues of safety or directions or letting parents know where I am.

   a) All outgoing calls will be made while the car is parked—not ever while moving—for the first six months.

   b) I will answer incoming calls from my parents only on the speaker phone (hands free).

2) We strongly discourage the use of the sound system in the car, at all, for the first 6 months of driving experience.

3) I promise not to have any passengers in the car while I am driving, other than my siblings or parents until _____ (six months). I will never transport more passengers than there are seat belts and will not drive the car until all passengers have buckled up

4) Should I get a traffic violation ticket, I agree to pay for the ticket (or, preferably, attend traffic school) as well as the difference in the insurance premium for as long as the premium is in effect. If the amount exceeds monies I have saved, I will work off the amount of money owed at minimum wage.

5) I agree to pay for damages that I incur not covered by insurance (deductible).

6) I will keep the car that I drive clean, inside and out, and be aware of its need for gas, oil, windshield washer fluid, etc. I will not bring the car home with the yellow "low gas" light lit.

7) Never let the gas tank go below half full.

8) I will use the car with the permission of my parents. If they have no knowledge of the fact that I am using it and to what purpose, I am in violation of this contract.

9) Should this car be given over to you for your exclusive use, this contract still applies and, in addition, you will be responsible for arranging and implementing (paying with your gas credit card) regular service for the car (check-ups, oil changes every 2,000 miles, tires, wipers, etc.).

10) AT NO TIME will I ever drink alcohol or do drugs and then drive. Nor will there be any alcohol, drugs, or cigarettes in the car at any time—even if it is friends who are doing it.

11) I will test my blood glucose level before beginning to drive the car each and every time I start to drive after a lapse of 2 hours since last being in the driver's role.

12) I will double check that I have rapid-acting glucose available in the car before I begin driving—each time I begin driving.

13) If I feel low or high, I will immediately pull off at the nearest safe spot, check, and call a parent while doing so.

I have read the above agreement and do sign this is accordance with the rules.

Signed,

Driver   Date

Parent   Parent

CHAPTER TEN

The Other "Big D"—Drinking and Diabetes

Since my daughter with diabetes was the second teen I'd raised, I knew ahead of time that assumptions such as my child would never drink alcohol while underage were not based in reality. And yet, the idea of her sneaking even a beer terrified me. Since I'd read all about how alcohol can impact blood sugars, I feared she would sneak her first drink and end up hurt, sick … or worse. My decision was to make sure she was safe. I wanted her to learn all about drinking at an early age, not to dissuade her (although the last thing I'd want to do is encourage her. Drinking and teens are not a good mix for many reasons). Rather, I wanted her to approach it with some smarts, some confidence, and total honesty with me. As a result, I know the first time my daughter drank an alcoholic *beverage. I know because she shared the entire experience with me the next morning. (It was kind of funny: her sipping a hard lemonade, her friends checking her blood sugars over and over and stressing all night about it. It was probably the opposite of a "wild time," although they felt like they'd been wild.) When she went off to college, far away from me, she knew how to manage alcohol and diabetes, what to do, what to drink and not to drink, and when to ask for help. Am I a bad mother for having allowed her to learn this under my watch? This I know: she's a smart girl who takes good care of herself and yes, she goes to frat parties, but always with a plan. She's safe. And for that, I'm glad of my decision.*

It is up to parents to make their own decisions on this issue, but one thing I believe: if you and your medical team are not at least talking about drinking and diabetes from the time a child reaches the teen years, you need to be. Education helps. That's my take.

It ranks up high in the fears parents have facing their children's teen years with diabetes: what if they want to drink? The first thing that needs to be said here is that the purchase or public possession of alcohol for anyone under 21 in the United States is illegal (this is not the case in other countries, so parents there cannot worry about that). It is your job to help your child want to stay within the law.

But it is also your role as a parent to make sure your child with diabetes is educated about alcohol and what impact it has on blood glucose. The child who does not know might be more tempted to try it without a plan. And the child who does know may be more willing to be honest with you, should he or she make an illegal choice or get into a dangerous situation with alcohol. Openness on this topic is a good idea, and not just a few weeks before your child leaves for college. Start young and help teens to understand that when they are the proper age, drinking is not prohibited with diabetes, and that if they do choose to disobey you now, they should know they can call you for help.

What Booze Does

Alcohol is processed by the liver, since it is a toxin, and the job of the liver (well, one of the jobs of the liver) is to process and remove toxins. When a liver is busy processing alcohol, it stops doing some other things, such as helping process and use your insulin. In short, this means that while your body is busy processing alcohol, your insulin hangs out in your body, which can make you go temporarily higher than you might usually expect from that amount of insulin.

Add this to the equation: it can take many, many hours for the body to process alcohol, which means that insulin is hanging out and waiting. And when it is finally "insulin's turn," it can hit hard, making you go low. The most common mistake a person uneducated in drinking makes is to see that high that comes a few hours into drinking and do an extra insulin correction. Then, hours later when the liver is back to paying attention to the insulin again, there's too much, and a crashing low can follow.

Sounds like you'd just be better off not drinking, you say? That's not how teens and young adults think. So instead, they need to learn how to manage drinking safely.

Knowing that they might be high when they come home is good information. When in college, they'll learn to not correct that high and, instead, wait it out for at least six hours or more. But with extra checks so as to avoid diabetic ketoacidosis (DKA). (It all sounds fun, doesn't it?) And here's where the honesty comes in: let's say your teen goes out and sneaks a few drinks. They come home, and you see that blood sugar is high. If a teen doesn't fess up to the drinking, he or she has to go along with you suggesting, and overseeing, a correction. If a teen feels safe enough to say "I drank, and this is what I drank," you can make an educated choice on what to do.

"Best Practices"?

So what's the best way to drink? Some hints:
- **Don't bolus for carbs.** In fact, people with diabetes who drink should look to either drink something with carbs (like beer or a mixer that is not sugar free), or eat while they drink. And they should be very slow in covering those carbs with insulin. Remember that alcohol makes one low. You need the carbs to balance that off even if it makes you high for a while.
- **Don't get falling-down drunk.** Period. And if you do, call for help immediately or encourage someone else to. Here's the thing: if you end up unconscious, even if it's "just from drinking," it's going to have to be treated as a diabetes emergency. Because who would know if it wasn't? And even if you are tipsy, you are going to lose your ability to reason about what you are doing and what you are eating and drinking. All dangerous. Teens need to realize that getting falling-down drunk for them is a crisis and

needs to be treated that way. Encourage them to—when they are old enough—drink responsibly.

- **Glucagon does not work when there is alcohol in the body.** This is important to know. The liver is busy, as we said, and that affects glucagon, too. So should a teen drink, have a low, and not be able to swallow food, the only options are honey, icing, glucose gels, or syrup in the mouth and/or a call to 911 for intravenous glucose. It is crucial for parents and teens to know this fact.
- **Avoid the "jungle juice."** Those giant punch bowls full of a fruity concoction that you cannot quite figure out? Not a good idea. Better to go with beer—so you know exactly what it is—or a drink you mix yourself.
  Teens tend to laugh at the idea of just drinking a spritzer in a fancy glass (not much of that on hand at a frat party). But beer is almost always available, and most adults with type 1 say it's a safer choice.
- **Have a buddy system.** This is a good idea for all teens, but more so for teens with diabetes. If you have had even a drink or two, you are not old enough or in control enough to be making decisions on a shot or a pump button. And you need a friend who is sober to not only drive you home, but hit your "home" speed dial if things go awry. Encourage your child not to drink—but to know he or she can have someone call you if you are needed.

In time, college teens (who do tend to drink) find a pattern that works for them, and a type of drink that works best for them, and tend to stick to it. In many cases, once the "excitement" of drinking wears down, young adults with diabetes decide that the hard work of drinking correctly with diabetes makes it not as much worth it.

Of course, if you tell your teen this now, he or she is only going to want to do it more. So talk it up. And expect their medical team to as well. In fact, a teen's medical team should start this discussion before you even feel it is necessary.

In the end, we don't want our teens to drink. But it's best that they understand the implications, know what action to take, and feel completely comfortable calling on an adult for help when needed.

CHAPTER ELEVEN

The Taste of Freedom

The following is a blog I wrote that ran in "Diabetes Mine" back in 2009. While our lives have changed so much for the better since then, the theme still rings true, and I believe that what I wrote is the perfect introduction to this chapter.

Walking into my kitchen to do one of the billion chores it seems I have to do every day of my life, I was stopped short by the emotion that overtook me when I noticed what was on the counter.

Used test strips. Three of them. Not in the trash, not put away. Now before you think I'm a neat freak, consider this: the surge of emotion I felt was pure, undiluted joy. Because the test strips littering my granite countertop were evidence of the most beautiful kind I could ever imagine.

They were evidence that my daughter was checking her blood sugar.

Why, you ask, would this send me so over the moon when she's had diabetes for 13 of her 18 years on this earth? When the total finger pricks she's done definitely number in the forty thousands? Because, you see, she's that truly puzzling soul: a teenage girl who has had diabetes for more than a decade. And while I struggle to get my head around it, that has meant for her—more times than not in the past five years—periods of seldom checking, ignoring blood sugars until they skyrocket to stomach-retching highs, and "forgetting" to bolus for snacks (and even meals sometimes), and a constant state of combined worry, anger, and sadness for me.

I tell you this because I think it's time that we all just stood up and admitted what is true in many homes: our teens—even the brightest, smartest, funniest, and most driven of them all—have a hard time dealing with the day-to-day demands of diabetes. I know firsthand. My daughter was the "model patient" for oh-so-many years.

So, one would think the idea of pricking her finger to check her blood sugar six or so times a day and then counting her carbs and pushing some buttons on her pump must not be such a big deal, right? It's just something one has to do, and that's that, correct?

Think again. Because diabetes is the one thing that trips

my daughter up. Constantly. It started the summer before she turned 13. I'd yelled across our club pool for her to check her blood sugar, and she just was not in the mood to do it. Instead, she tried something "new." She fiddled with her meter for a bit and then yelled back across the pool to me, "I'm 173!" I nodded, reminded her to correct, jotted it down in her color-coded logbook, and went on with my day.

She told me months later that that was her turning point: the moment she tasted the "drug" she'd struggled with for years. That drug is called freedom. That day, she realized that I trusted her so much, she could pretty much do or not do whatever she wanted. The idea of not checking was so delicious, she still says today she thinks she must know what drug addicts feel like when they try to detox. She skipped testing more and more. By fall, she started skipping insulin doses, too. And as she told me after she landed in the ICU and almost died, as sick as it made her feel physically, the emotional high of DENYING diabetes any power in her life (and yes, I do see the irony here) made that horrid feeling all worth the while.

So the ICU trip was my wake-up call. It all came clear; she fessed up. I worked at being more in her face and actually looking at the meter and the pump. Her A1C came down. And by the next summer, I was back to being the trusting mom again. She never did land in the ICU again, but her blood sugars have suffered. She seemed to have two good weeks of doing what she should, and then she'd fall apart again. As she grew older and was not with me as often, it became easier and easier for her to hide her secret. And as much as she intellectually knew what she was doing was wrong, the addiction held tight. After a particularly jarring A1C one year, she tried to explain her struggle to me.

"It's like I go to bed at night and I say, 'Tomorrow morning I'm going to wake up and start new and do what I am supposed to do. I'm going to check regularly and take my insulin. I'm going to bolus every time I eat. And starting tomorrow, it will be fine.' But then I wake up and I just cannot do it, Mom. Does that make any sense?"

Ummmm. That explains the success of the Weight Watchers program. We mere humans want to do right and start fresh. We know well what we have to do, and yet ... we stumble. Of course I understood. But the thing was: it's her life she's messing with. Each time she stumbled again, my heart hurt more.

I could never admit any of this to just about anyone, either. My non-diabetes-world friends would say something like, "Well, isn't it just a matter of discipline?" Or, "Well, you need to just take control!" And even my diabetes-world friends would judge. Everyone's kids seem to have an A1C of 6.3. None of them mind checking, and they all fully understand why they should change out their site every three days even if it still seems pretty good (or so they all say). I'm the only bad mom. My daughter is the only bad diabetic. That's what I thought.

Until I started to be honest about it. Lauren spoke before Congress about her struggles, and the line of people waiting to talk to her afterward stretched out seemingly forever. There were kids who had done the same thing and not admitted it, parents who feared their children were doing the same, parents who wanted to figure out how to keep their kids from doing it, or kids saying "OMG. You totally told my tale." Then I started to hint to D-world friends that all was not ducky in our house. A few brave souls reached out to me and told me —privately—that they, too, were struggling with their teens. Still, I sit here today a bit shamed as I write this.

After all, I am my daughter's protector. I am her defensive linebacker. How could I let anything bad come her way? I mean, diabetes? I could not block that. But complications? That's on my watch. Good Lord.

But here is the thing: I really believe that by addressing this openly, we are going to help millions of people and even save billions of dollars. What if there was no shame attached to a teen with diabetes rebelling? What if it was no different from, say, admitting your kid skipped doing homework and got a zero on something (what kid hasn't done that once)?

What if instead of hiding in shame, teens—and parents of teens—had an open forum to discuss their situation and find ways to make things better? It's time for the noncompliant teen and his or her parent to come out of the closet.

The sad thing is this: some mom (or dad) out there with an eight-year-old with diabetes is going to read this and cluck her (or his) tongue and say, "I'm glad I didn't raise my kid that way. I'm glad my child doesn't do that." She's going to be smug; she's not going to agree. I know this because I was that mom. I had it all figured out. And look where that smugness landed us. So if that person is you, I don't want to hear it. But should you ever need support and understanding if you face this, I'll be here for you.

My daughter is doing better this week; thus the test strips littering my countertop. Her last endo appointment was a nightmare. Her A1C came up high, and her endo told her, in no uncertain terms, something that had been in the back of my head: if she does not change her ways and prove herself, she will not be heading off to the amazing college so far away that we've put a deposit on for her.

I hate that while other kids are stressing over roommates, she is figuring out how to break years of difficult diabetes struggles. I despise that she really does have to take this on the right way once and for all. But, as I smile through tears at the litter on the counter, I feel overwhelming hope. I adore my daughter. She's strong, smart, funny, and good at heart. She can do it. And the best thing I can do for her is admit that it's hard, help her try, understand when she slips up, and work hard for that elusive better way of life for her down the road.

Teens and What Freedom Means

Remember when all they wanted to do was hang out with you, please you, and be a part of your life? For all teens—not just teens with diabetes—a big part of their "job" in growing up now is working toward independence. While those days of wanting to be a positive center of your world were delightful, now they have a new focus: their social world and all it entails. And for the most part, it does not include you.

As harsh as that may sound, this is actually a crucial time for all teens to begin forging ahead toward their own identities, social groups, and lives. In fact, while you have long been the guiding light for all your child needs to learn and understand, even that is shifting now. In these years, peer relationships actually become the proving ground where they learn about social and cultural norms. In other words, it's where they figure out how to fit in, relate, and succeed in the world.

So when your teen begins pushing away from you and looking for freedom, that's almost instinctual. The problem is, teens have all the motor skills they need to succeed in life mastered (hand-eye coordination, writing, running and walking safely, etc.). What they still don't quite have down are the intellectual skills needed to fare well in life. Which sets all teens and parents up for a challenging push-pull: the teen wants to be left to his or her own devices, since he or she feels confident about knowing it all. Parents want to hold tight to the control they've had all their child's life to date. Somewhere in the middle is the answer.

For all teens, freedom means being able to feel like they can "do their own thing" without their parents breathing down their necks. And in some ways, parents can help teens do this while safe. Letting them go to the beach for the day, for instance, when in the past you'd always insist on a parent being along, is an appropriate step toward freedom. Where you once needed to know everyone they were with and every moment's plan, in the teen years you can live with "I'll be at the North Beach until 3 p.m. We are not going anywhere else."

Freedom may mean, too, backing off on nagging about homework and schoolwork (although there can still be consequences if they don't perform to the standard you require). Freedom can mean they hang out with kids you might not know as well as you knew their grade school playgroup friends. These steps help a teen feel somewhat free, while not moving to the point of danger (Dangerous would be saying, "You can go sleep over a house where I don't know the parents for an entire weekend, and I won't check on you"). But baby steps toward making them feel unencumbered by you while still safe is the right process. That's for all teens.

Now, when you layer diabetes on top of that, it's a whole different level of concern, worry, and, yes, possibilities of danger. That means, like so many other things, parents of teens with diabetes must work hard to help their teens taste freedom while not letting them crash and burn.

Free Will and Daily Diabetes Dare: Not Always in Harmony

What does freedom mean to a teen with diabetes? Teens with

diabetes basically help run a life support system every minute of every day of their lives. Even when they were little and you were doing it all, they were there to witness it, feel it, and experience it. That's a lot of connection: to parents, to medical teams, to a disease, and to a lifestyle they may very well wish they could wave away.

That's why freedom, in the mind of the teen with diabetes, can get confusing. Sure, teens want freedom from having to talk about diabetes with parents and doctors and the rest of the world over and over and over. Sure, they want freedom to make their own decisions on what to eat and when to eat and how to handle it diabetes-wise. But often, in their mind, freedom becomes something more: a move toward partial or total disregard of anything diabetes related.

Teens will do things like skip checks, skip doses, and lie about it all, just to be "free" of it (see chapter 12 for more details on how to spot this and what to do). The irony, most teens will tell you when they sit and think about it, is this: not taking care of their diabetes to be "free" of it actually makes them feel worse (sick from highs or lows; tired from lack of sleep from having to get up to go to the bathroom, and more). And yet, the pull is almost irresistible to some.

> ### Check Your Own Psyche First
>
> Particularly if your child has had diabetes for a long time, you need to think about how you are feeling at this time. Parental burnout often comes at the same time as teen pushback. And now is not the time for you to step completely back. Make sure you are doing all you can for yourself at this time.

So is there anything a parent can do to help teens feel they have some freedom in all of this? There are steps you can consider, but they don't always work.

First, it needs to be said: teens should not be 100 percent on their own in their diabetes care, no matter what they may think or feel. While it is a time to begin moving toward true freedom, that should only be done with some parental supervision. Even if teens say they resent this, deep down they do not. And in the long run, when they truly are ready to be completely independent, this time with you still somewhat involved will have helped them.

But you can take some steps even from a somewhat early age to help them begin to feel some freedom. Some to consider (and discuss with your child's medical team):

- Consider letting teens help shape their diabetes plans. This might mean compromise from what you've always expected, but it could also mean that they feel like it's their plan and not one forced on them. For instance, they may feel they can get by on fewer checks. If their team agrees, you should agree.

- Work toward a place of not asking all the time. It's been said before in this book but cannot be said enough: we parents are very bad at *not* thinking of diabetes first when we see our children before or after school. Try not to ask, and you may help them not feel it's something they constantly need to escape. Remember, it's not always the diabetes. Kids do poorly on tests. And get cranky. And are thirsty. It's not always the diabetes.

- Make it easier for them. Ask your teen what you can do to make life with diabetes easier. Filling pump reservoirs when needed? Checking a teen's bag to make sure strips are included without commenting on it? Compiling a list of carb counts for meals teens tend to eat when out with their friends and inputting it into their smartphones? Whatever they want or agree to when you suggest, promise to have it done so they have less to think about.

Of course, much of this means adapting your own expectations. This could mean doing things in a way that you would not choose. And again, if your teen's medical team is onboard, your job as a parent is to try to adapt your expectations to fit with what your teen and their medical team have agreed upon. Not easy for a parent who worries about lows and highs and the long term with diabetes. But if you trust your teen's team and they are part of the plan, the best thing you can do is work with it, for the good of your child.

When a Teen's Attitude Means Trouble

So what if teens see freedom as diabetes being none of your business, or meaning that they can eat what they want when they want without taking insulin if they are not in the mood, or that they can totally ignore their diabetes?

This is a difficult situation that requires professional help, patience, and time. We discuss details of burnout in chapter 12, but if your teen is choosing to ignore diabetes care, you'll need to first and foremost make sure he or she is safe. This might mean, as much as it hurts them, taking some freedom away.

But only to a point. For instance, if a teen takes shots or boluses from a pump on his or her own, you might need to insist that at least twice each day—in the morning and at night—you see the insulin go into his or her body. And you also might need to witness at least one blood glucose reading per day, so you know it actually happened.

It's not advised to take away freedoms that have nothing to do with diabetes. For instance, telling teens they cannot go to the homecoming dance because they have not been following their diabetes plan does not make sense. Homecoming has nothing to do with diabetes. Nor do you want to take away the very activities that bring them joy, such as sports or a job outside the home. While you do need to remind them over and over and over that taking care of their diabetes only makes those joyful things better, removing them might push your child toward full-on resentment and even depression.

Some things are fair game for punishment, though. Driving is at the top of the list. We devoted a chapter to this, but remember, if a teen does not do what is required by diabetes behind the wheel, he or she should not be allowed to drive. Period.

So what if you are at the point where you are concerned about your child's immediate safety and long-term health? It can be both frustrating and terrifying for parents to witness their children abandon their daily care. This is discussed more in chapter 12.

The best hope you can have is keeping an honest and open conversation about how your teen feels and what freedoms he or she might desire. And while you will have to say "no" to some requests (just as parents of all teens have to), sometimes you can help teens feel like they've won some new freedom. That might just help through this challenging and confusing time.

CHAPTER TWELVE

Burnout, Rebellion, and Other Emotional Challenges

My daughter was the model diabetes patient for years and years. But somewhere in the middle of the teen years, it all took its toll. Burnout hit, and hit hard. I tried to get her to come around to realizing that the best power she would have over diabetes would be to not let it make her feel physically and mentally drained, but for some time she just could not come around to that. And we struggled. It took me a long time even to understand that she was burning out, and it took even longer to help bring her back on a road to wellness. But we learned a lot.

I wrote her a letter one day, and I said this:
This does not make it fair. Just because you CAN face all this down, you should not have to. But for now, it's here and you

must. I wish I could make it go away. I've tried throwing money at it, screaming at rallies at it, advocating the heck out of it. But diabetes is still here. So what are we to do?

Because like it or not, this challenge is yours. I can support you. I can love you beyond anything imaginable. But I cannot "do" diabetes for you like I could when you were little. I hope you know you are not alone. Really cool people, some you know quite well, have been down this road. They've struggled. They've fought it and ignored it and tried to deny it. They've worried about their future but still not had the strength to take charge. Then they've gotten up, brushed themselves off, and gone back at it again.

I wish with all my heart I could change all this. But it seems, for now, I cannot. So I have to ask you to do what is totally unfair and just be the strongest young woman alive. Is that so much to ask (tee hee)? Reach out to those who have been there. Talk to those who are there now like you. Go at it one day at a time, or one hour at a time. Whatever works. Find a way. Get up on your knees and smack the heck out of it. Use the tools we have to beat it down for now. Ask for more tools, reach out for more help. We will find you whatever you need to get by (even if it is yet another Vera Bradley bag to make carrying supplies all the more fun). No way it is easy. No way is it foolproof.

But you are the strongest young woman I know. Diabetes

sucks, but don't let it suck all the awesomeness out of you.

I wish I could say those words instantly cured the burnout, but they did not. We spent a lot of time working on things, and then, a year later, success. As suddenly as it all began, it all seemed to come around. And what she told me about it, after a positive appointment with her new endo she loved, was this:

"You know, great new endo or not, at the end of the day it really is what he told me from the start: this has to come from me. This is about me. This is my diabetes, my life, my choice. And I've finally realized that. That's why I'm doing so much better."

I hope this chapter helps you keep an eye out for possible burnout, take action, and help your teen to avoid it or at least recover as quickly as possible. Burnout can take years to overcome. But I'm happy to say overcome my daughter did. So, too, can all.

We all raise our children to do the right things—or at least we perceive that we do. With diabetes, this is no different. We want our children to be responsible but not overwhelmed, smart but not consumed by it. We work over the years (or the months in the case of a newly diagnosed teen) to help them know how to handle all this and how to use our support. And yet, life with T1D onboard can be overwhelming to even the most "together" of teens. In fact, teens that seem to juggle a lot with ease (grades, sports, a part-time job or a club, helping at home, and more) can be particularly susceptible to burnout—and even to rebellion. After all, they have the daunting combination of a lot to manage and an image they feel they need to uphold. They don't want to let anyone down, and so they take more and more on themselves. And when they cannot handle it, they hide it rather than admit it.

This is why more than one parent has been nearly blindsided by a child's diabetes burnout.

The teen with additional struggles (and most teens today have them)—from dealing with parental divorce to bending to peer pressure to getting involved with illegal activities and more—that teen's journey to burnout and/or rebellion can be even rockier. (I talk details about dangerous situations in chapter 13.) Often, struggles with such non-diabetes issues lead a teen to give up or burn out on diabetes, or to just say, "To heck with it." It all can seem overwhelming and, often, diabetes care is the first to be tossed aside.

So what's a parent to do?

This is what you need to understand first: burning out, and even rebelling, is not an act of aggression; it is more an act of desperation. Kids—and adults—get sick of the constant attention diabetes demands. One adult with type 1 once said he would "pay $10,000 for just one day off from diabetes." Imagine teens, whose minds are not fully formed yet, and what they would "pay" to feel as if they were "getting a day off." The feeling of a long-time high blood sugar can suddenly become tempting, even welcome. The danger of a low from not checking disappears. The need to carefully count the carbs on your plate evaporates. Just that, ignoring the needs of diabetes itself can become intoxicating.

The first step is to never assume it won't happen, no matter how smooth a path you've laid down for your teen. Be vigilant, look for the signs and never, ever say "Not my child." True, your child could sail through the teen years without burnout. But by not assuming he or she will avoid it, you may just catch the signs before it gets to a critical point.

Why Does It Happen?

Burnout and rebellion hit all kinds of teens from all kinds of families. If your child faces some of this, it is not because you are a bad parent and others are good; it's just the way your teen is dealing with it (or not dealing).

Some people think kids who are diagnosed at a young age tend to hit burnout more than those who come to this diabetes life later. It could make sense that the child who has had to face daily diabetes care for a decade or longer might get sick of it all. It could also be the case that parents of children who have had diabetes for a long time tend to trust their children more; after all, diabetes care has been a part of your lives for so long, you as a parent can begin to take for granted that it all just happens.

It is also believed that teens who can have days of particularly proficient plan compliance and still see blood sugars soar or plummet (thank you, hormones) can get to a point of feeling like "Well, what's the point?" If they try their hardest and still see results they don't particularly enjoy, that can lead to a feeling of defeat, emotional exhaustion, and, eventually, just not wanting to try anymore. Parents can—without meaning to—add to the teen's negative feelings about blood checking by questioning or criticizing blood glucose values more than they praise the teen for the act of checking. When BG checking becomes burdened down with negative feelings and is no longer about getting helpful information, burnout can develop. And most parents don't even realize they are doing it. Saying something as simple as "Why were you high again?" can come off as criticism to a teen. The less you can use any judgmental tone in talking about it, the better. For instance, instead of saying "Why were you high?" you could say "I see you were high. I hope that did not make you feel sick." And see what conversation comes from that.

And some teens just plain hit a point of having had enough of it. It's not hard to understand: imagine having something you absolutely have to do many times a day, forever and ever. It's daunting to the adult mind. Imagine what it does to the teen mind. Even the teen only a year into this can just feel beaten down. And turning away from it becomes a way to escape, although ironically, it's not escaping at all.

Signs of Burnout and Rebellion

It would be nice if there were some kind of visible warning that a teen was struggling with daily care. But it's not like high blood sugars or unchecked blood sugars make your fingernails change color. Instead, parents are left looking for clues, and often, missing clues that in hindsight seemed to be right in front of them. In fact, clues can be so thoroughly overlooked that often a greatly elevated A1C is the parent's first hint that things are not as they seem (and this can be confusing, too, since most teens experience an increase in A1C values due to things like hormones and growth spurts impacting blood glucose values). There are, however, some common things parents can keep an eye out for. If you see any of these, it may not mean your child is struggling. But it does mean you should consider it and look for more signs, as well as talk with your child and the medical team. Some signs include:

- **Skipped blood checks.** There may be excuses that seem to make sense (I forgot my meter. I didn't have time. My strips ran out. The battery was dead.). If you see it happening more and more, consider that your child may be looking for excuses for a blood check he or she simply did not do (I address lying later in this chapter). Some teens will go as far as to "lose a meter" so parents won't know they've not been checking.

- **Skipped doses.** For many of the same reasons as above. When it happens more and more, consider the possibility that the teen just plain did not want to do it.
- **More and more unexplained highs or lows.** If you suddenly notice teens are spiking way more often, needing to change out pump sites or do large corrections, even though you cannot rule out the possible "real" reasons (such as a malfunctioning pump, a need for ratio changes, or a need for different injection sites), you may want to consider the possibility that your child might not be doing what he or she claims to be doing, and is looking for help only when it's necessary, such as when feeling sick from a high. If your "parent gut" starts telling you, "This is strange," you may want to consider the possibility that it's not happening for the reasons your teen claims.
- **Secrecy.** If teens never want you to see their pump settings, their meter results, or their bottle of test strips, take notice. Of course, teens are not above doing things like throwing out unused strips, pumping insulin through tubing while not connected (so the pump will read as if a bolus was done), and, sigh, using control solution to do fake checks on a meter. In fact, if you suddenly notice that the control solution is being used or is out in places you don't expect it to be, take notice as well.

BURNOUT FROM A TEEN PERSPECTIVE

The teenage years are hard for anyone growing up, but having diabetes thrown into the mix just makes everything a hundred times more complicated. It all started for me around the age of thirteen, or seventh grade. I'd had diabetes for about seven years at that point. I remember the first time I lied about checking my blood to my mom. She had asked me what I was when I checked, and I said "120" without any hesitation. She didn't question it, and I knew she wasn't going to any time soon. She trusted me. But I had totally made that number up.

I continued to lie about my numbers and then began to lie about taking my insulin. After a few months, I ended up in the ICU in DKA. You would think that this would be a wakeup call to a teenager, maybe to change my ways and never lie about my diabetes again. Well, my habits did change for the better, but not for long. After a few months, I was back into my old habits again.

This is because teenagers *don't think about things that are happening far in the future*. I had countless people and doctors telling me "your kidneys could fail in ten years if you keep this up" or "blindness occurs in people with diabetes who don't excel in taking care of themselves." The way that I looked at it was, nothing *that horrible* had happened to me yet, and I would rather focus on my social life than worry about things that are so far away in the future that I cannot even begin to picture them. In other words, the threats did not work because I did not care, and I did not believe they applied to me. The times I did start to think about it, I felt more like "Well, I guess I've already ruined myself" more than "I can stop this and help myself." All those things did was mess with my head, if you ask me.

That being said, I did want to change my habits. I obviously didn't like feeling horrible all the time, and I wanted to live a long, healthy life, but I just couldn't make myself care about it for longer than a week at a time. Promising myself that I would check my blood five times or more a day every day when I had barely been checking at all was setting myself up to fail. I would try so hard to make it happen, and I always failed. I spent many nights crying in my room, wishing I could just do it right. Diabetes just wasn't my top priority.

After multiple endocrinologists and five years of my life struggling with taking care of myself, I finally ended up with an endocrinologist who *got what I was going through*.

He told me to set short-term goals, like to check my blood when I wake up and when I go to bed. We would work on checking more after I get those two checks down. Eventually my A1C came down, and taking care of myself got easier for me. If I could go back to when I was in the "burnout" stage, I would have probably have focused more on setting smaller goals for myself. Such as, "I will check my blood every time I eat today," or "I will give myself my insulin before I eat today."

Little things are much easier to follow than a goal of "I will take care of myself." Saying that type of thing to yourself as a teenager, or telling a teenager to do that, is

continued on next page

ultimately a setup for failure. It was like by setting a vague goal like "I will take care of myself," the minute I did one thing wrong (like skip a check or a bolus), in my mind, I had already failed. So I'd give up. I think if I had known—and my mom had known—to set those smaller goals back then, I *might* have turned it around faster.

Then again, I was a teenager, and who knows? But I do know that the one thing I'd tell parents of teens who are having a hard time is to help them pick some small things they can feel successful with. Instead of saying something like "You have to check six times a day," find a way to help them have a smaller goal. And don't threaten or nag. It did me no good at all.

I also think it is good for teens to hear that they are *not* heading toward a certain terrible future (kidney failure, etc.). At our first appointment, my adult doctor told me, "You do know that you are going to be fine and you have not destroyed your body, right?" It was such a relief, and actually motivated me to take better care.

I'm glad my mother stuck by me in those hard years, and I'm really glad she let me move to a doctor who thought the way my new doctor did. I'm so much better now. And I now actually know that when I make up a number, the only one I'm lying to is myself.

Lauren Stanford

These are all hints that parents may need to pay closer attention to what is going on with their teens, which is a challenge in itself, since teens spend so much time away from us. It's a challenge, too, because communication with teens can be touchy at best. When they are looking to not interact, they can lash out as an attempt to either stop us from trying or to put up a smokescreen to change the topic. You started with, "Gosh, have you not been checking?" And the teen's huffy retort changed it to, "Don't talk to me like that." These teens are clever. But hey, we raised them, right?

Lying: The Big One

Intertwined in almost all of this is the theme of lying. Teens who are looking to avoid their diabetes self-care (as well as many other things) will resort to lying and sneaking around, not just to get away with it, but to avoid it. Some teens are so adept at their lying that parents are left thinking: Gosh, if they used that power for good, they could save the world! Easy to laugh now, but when you are in the middle of it, it's more than hard.

For the act of lying hurts most parents, and hurts them to the core. We raise our children to learn about trust and honesty. When they lie, we not only feel hurt and betrayed; we feel we've failed. It is important to look deep at the lying and understand where it comes from and what to do about it. It does not make it right, but it can make it easier to understand.

First of all, most lies when it comes to diabetes are not done to be evil or bad. Rather, most teens just don't want to disappoint us. They are like big toddlers in that way. They practice "magical thinking." If they say it is true enough times, that will make it true. Part of their burnout is wishing their diabetes away; lying about it to you is wishing away that they've been wishing it away.

So let's say your teen has been lying about how often he or she is checking. How do you solve the problem? Here's a somewhat simple tip: just don't ask.

What was that? Wouldn't not asking mean your child could just run amuck? Well, not if you "don't ask" the right way. Instead of asking, just look at the meter. Because here's the thing: other than when kids manipulate them, meters don't lie.

So a good idea for parents is to proactively start this practice before you even consider there may be signs of burnout or rebellion. Start the habit of looking at the meter every day at the same time (after dinner can be a good time; kids are usually doing homework and almost the entire day is logged at that point). What you see is what happened (or did not happen) that day. Now, the challenge for you as a parent is how you react to that.

Because if your child did not lie and you simply saw that a check or two was missing or numbers were particularly high or low and you did not know, the issue is no longer about lying. And remember: we as parents are not supposed to get angry or upset at numbers, or, really, even at teens not completing all their daily diabetes tasks. Rather, we are supposed to assess, give input, help fix in the moment, and then move on with a next-steps plan. It all sounds so basic on paper, doesn't it?

So instead of saying to your teen, "You did not check all day today at school!" you should say, "I see you were not able to check today. Is there something we can do to help you? And, can you check now so we can correct if needed?" The idea is to take away the opportunity for the teen to lie, while demonstrating to your teen that you can be rational when things do not go as planned.

Will it stop teens from lying? Maybe not, but it will plant the seed that even when things don't go well, everything can be worked out. After all, there is no going backward in diabetes. We must always move forward.

Parents and teens also have the option today of smartphone apps that share meter results. You may want to consider this and include your teen in the discussion. But like checking the meter each evening, this will involve your showing some restraint even when things do not look the way you'd prefer them to.

There are times, however, when lying must be dealt with. For instance, if a teen claims to have checked before driving and did not, this is a situation where privileges should be taken away. Since driving without knowing what your blood sugar is can be dangerous not only for your teen but for everyone else on the road, teens must obey that rule.

That said, it might not be the same situation if a teen lied about checking after school, and you said the teen could not go to the school dance. One does not match the other.

And what of the kind of lie that takes premeditation, such as using control solution to fake a glucose check? First, unless you catch your teen red-handed, it can be dangerous to accuse. So if you suspect this may be happening, the best solution is to remove the tools teens can use to create the lie. Take all control solution and keep it where your teen cannot get at it. You might also want to plant a seed in your teen's head that you know it can happen—something like "David's mom found out he used control solution for a check. Have you ever heard of such a thing?"

Parents, for the most part, want to punish teens for lying, and for good reason: being honest is a trait we want to make sure our children have. But with diabetes issues, we must tread carefully and make sure our actions are for the best.

One question you will need to ask yourself if you see burnout in your child is this: is this burnout or depression? In the following chapter, we discuss depression at length.

Rebellion

You follow all this carefully, making sure you are treading lightly yet still doing your best to keep your teen safe. But the teen just pushes back more. In time, your teen flat-out refuses to do what he or she needs to do. Now what steps can a parent take?

Counseling is the first thought, and that means for your teen as well as for you. This life with diabetes is not an easy one. Being a teen in this century is not easy. Sometimes when the two collide, it can mean danger. It is up to you, at the end of the day, to keep your teen safe. And if getting extra help moves you toward that, so be it.

You can first talk to your child's endo team. If they have a social worker on the team, that person, along with the CDE and/or endo, may be able to shed light on your situation. Is it as worrisome as you suspect? Listen to the team: they've seen all this before. They may have a counselor to suggest, and they may not. If they do, consider trying that counselor first. In a perfect world, you'll find a counselor who understands teens, burnout, rebellion, and type 1 diabetes. That said, if you cannot find this, work on finding a counselor to whom your child can relate, and take it from there. If the counselor has no experience with a teen with type 1, you'll need to make sure any advice the counselor gives your teen is safe and proper. Ask your child's endocrine team to help you with this, via e-mails, letters, or other communication with the counselor.

Important to consider, too, is compromise. This is a hard one for parents to swallow, but it may be time for your teen, along with the medical team, to make the main decisions on the daily care plan. Let's say you've always liked your teen to do eight checks a day, three in school (and this is just an example, not a suggestion). What if your teen, along with his or her medical team, decides that five checks a day (or four), with one at school, would work well?

As long as the medical team is onboard, giving teens this kind of power may help them feel like they do have some control, like they can listen to their own feelings and then find a positive way to make changes and adjustments that just make living with diabetes less invasive.

Your Own Burnout and Rebellion

The other twist here is somewhat ironic: at a point in your child's life when he or she may need you on your "diabetes A game" the most, you may just be completely burned out yourself.

Raising a child with diabetes is all-consuming. If you are an at-home parent, a full-time working parent, a part-time custodial parent, or some other kind of parent, it is nearly impossible to clear diabetes from your mind. From the script refills to fighting with insurance to planning on the medical appointments to making room in the butter compartment for all the insulin to knowing the carb count to every food on earth to the constant worry ... it can wear you down.

And for parents, the easiest way to deal with burnout is usually to pass on the bulk of the care to your child, and to trust the child so that you can breathe a bit. Even if you don't do it consciously, it's an easy trap to fall into.

When you add to that the fact that often teens are not, ahem, so nice to their parents, you might feel a streak of rebellion yourself. ("Oh, he thinks he's so smart; let him deal with it!" might go through your mind.)

The best thing parents can do to help their children avoid burnout is to avoid burning out themselves first. Take proactive steps. Take care of yourself so you can be up to helping your teen through this hard time, and so you can be on your toes to notice little hints that your teen needs extra help.

How, you ask, can you take care of yourself when you have so much to do to take care of others, including your child with diabetes? The old airplane flight instruction is the classic reason: give yourself oxygen first so you can be strong enough to help others. This is what you must do here.

But how? Here are some suggestions to start as early as you can. And do *not* feel guilty about them. You must be strong to keep your child strong, and to have the power to help your child when he or she is weak.

- **Get help.** If you are like most parents of kids with diabetes, you don't have a lot of backup help with your child and his or her needs. It's time to reach out to a friend or family member and just ask that person to get educated to give you a day off—even once a month. You might be surprised how often someone is willing. And educating the helper is possible, even if it takes time. Having a comrade whom you can call and to whom you can say, "I need to go overnight to a hotel just to breathe" can be a great help. True, your child cannot take a break from diabetes, but you can, and it can help you regroup to help them.
- **Professional help.** Consider counseling, even as a preventive measure. You have faced a lot and will face a lot. Some perspective and a place to talk things out can help a lot.
- **Pamper yourself.** If you can afford spa time, take it. If you cannot, take a long walk or treat yourself to a night once a week at the local library where you just read in peace. Or join some kind of club that has nothing to do with diabetes, and don't talk about diabetes there. Your head and soul will appreciate it.

By taking care of yourself, you can be better ready to stand on guard and help your child when he or she may need it most.

When to Say "When"

How do you know when your child is in true danger and you need to take more action? Dangerous situations are discussed in the next chapter. As far as burnout and rebellion go, stay in contact with your child's medical team and keep them up to date on what is going on. They can help you see when you might need to take more drastic action, or when, as is the case most of the time, you need to just provide support, guidance, a safety net, and patience.

Because the good news is this: Teens grow to be adults. And believe it or not, they really are listening to you. When their brain grows to use what they've heard, you'll see your hard work was worth it.

CHAPTER THIRTEEN

Depression and Diabetes

Thankfully, we have yet to have dealt with any of the *truly dangerous situations that can pop up around life with type 1 diabetes. I hope we never have to. But we've been alongside many friends who have. Watching dear friends grapple with not just depression but depression and diabetes, or not just an eating disorder but one with insulin in the mix, or not just drug abuse but drug abuse when you are dependent on a constant medical plan to keep you alive; well, it's beyond frightening. I am thankful we have avoided these issues (so far). But I never did—and never will—wear blinders. As difficult as it is to imagine, as frightening as it is to absorb, we parents simply must read the "hard parts." At worst, we need to be on the ready should certain situations arise. At best, we need to be prepared even if we never use any of the knowledge. This chapter touches on some of the more common dangerous situations. We hope you don't need it now and don't need it later. But we all need to know. Just in case.*

The teen years can be littered with sticky, frightening, and sometimes truly dangerous situations. There is no kidding around about dangerous situations and our teens with type 1 diabetes. From depression to drug abuse to "diabulimia" (which is not its real name; we'll get into that in this chapter), teens with diabetes may not just have to grapple with situations that would be dangerous to anyone; they may have to do the grappling with diabetes onboard, which makes it all the more worrisome. The best thing parents can do is understand the dynamics behind each situation, stay on guard for signs, hope for the best, and, as always, never, ever say, "It won't happen to us."

Depression

According to a study published by the Joslin Diabetes Center, the occurrence of depression in teens with diabetes is double that of the occurrence in teens without diabetes (*care.diabetes journals.org/content/29/6/1389.full*). This means parents of teens with diabetes, and preteens as well, need to think ahead, not just knowing signs but understanding what can lead to depression with diabetes onboard.

The basic underlying reason is simple, and it's hard not to know it: type 1 diabetes is hard. The daily—even sometimes hourly—requirements on teens can be overwhelming. And since teens struggle with so much in life in general—from peer pressure to self-image to the pressure to succeed—the overlay of what diabetes demands can easily become "the straw that breaks the camel's back." In other words, type 1 diabetes is not thought to cause depression in a biological way, but it is believed to contribute to depression due to the lifestyle aspects and the stress that living with diabetes can bring.

But here's the rub: teens can be moody, oversensitive, emotional creatures without depression or diabetes onboard. So how is a parent to know when it's whining and complaining and when it's something more serious? Understanding the signs and symptoms can help you separate the "moody teen stomping to room" syndrome from a true depressive situation you need to handle. Some symptoms include:

- **Loss of pleasure.** Does your teen no longer take pleasure in situations and events they used to enjoy? It's important to clarify this: if your teen no longer enjoys going to the movies with just you, that might just be because parents are boring. But if your teen no longer enjoys going to the movies—or other places—with most anyone, that could be a hint at an underlying issue.
- **Changes in sleep patterns.** Is your teen suddenly restless at night and unable to sleep? Or sleeping a ridiculous amount of time? Again, teens change their sleep patterns anyway. They stay up late online or studying; they snooze on weekends longer than you can imagine. But if you see a remarkable change, one that is interfering with their ability to focus and contribute (be it from sleeping too much or from exhaustion from inability to sleep a solid night), that could be a hint as well.
- **Changes in appetite.** Loss of appetite and/or the inability to enjoy a meal can be a sign of depression. We'll talk

about eating disorders later in this chapter.

- **Difficulty concentrating.** Again, teens have a lot going on in their lives and can be distracted often. But if your teen is unable to focus on tasks such as homework or chores, or has trouble even focusing on a TV show with the family, you may take that as a possible hint.
- **Talk of self-harm or self-hate.** Of course this is an obvious sign. And while teens can be prone to melodrama, such talk cannot be ignored and should be investigated.
- **Slack in or elimination of daily diabetes care routine.** Teens with diabetes tend to just give up. Burnout can lead to depression, but it does not necessarily mean your teen is depressed. But if your teen does suffer burnout and begins to not take care of his or her diabetes, you'll need to consider depression as a possibility.

Parents who see more than one of these signs should take action, if just to be sure your child is not suffering from depression.

What to do? First, you'll need to rule out physical reasons. It's most likely that your child's annual blood work includes thyroid tests. Ask your child's medical team when the last one was taken and if they feel another is needed. Sometimes, an issue with the thyroid can impact mood.

Once that is eliminated as a possibility, you'll need to consider counseling and even, if warranted and decided upon by doctors, medical intervention. As discussed with burnout, you'll want to find a therapist or psychiatrist who understands type 1 diabetes and teens, or at the least is willing to learn more about it. As with depression and diabetes, there can be a vicious circle. Teens feel depressed and overwhelmed and think, "What's the use? Even if I try hard at diabetes care I never get 'better.'" Or they think, "I'm just going to get complications anyway. Why bother?" They cut back on their daily care and begin to experience more highs or lows. This in turn makes them feel physically worse and more tired, which can lead to feeling more depressed about diabetes. How does a parent combat that? With support and information.

Prevention First

As discussed earlier in this book, teens may act as if they want to be independent in their care. But the longer you can hold some control (and therefore support) for them, the less the chance of burnout, overwhelmed feelings, and, yes, even depression. The earlier you can remember to not praise them for independence and to keep supporting them in every way you can, the better off they will be.

And arm them with information. The plain truth is that the death sentence that came with type 1 diabetes even just a few decades ago is no longer the case. Remember, your teen may not be hearing that good news out there in the world where people say, well, stupid things. It is your job as a parent to educate your child on what the reality is today. While you don't want to undersell the need for teens to

> ### Practice "Strewing"
>
> What, you ask, is strewing? Strewing is leaving things around for teens to pick up and read on their own. A positive story on long-term life with diabetes. A story on how to deal with alcohol and diabetes. Rather than say "read this," just leave it where they can find it. You can even try links on your Facebook page if your teen is your friend. Strewing allows them to "discover it" on their own.

keep up with their daily care, you do want to assure them that so long as they do a relatively decent job of it, chances are they will not die young or face complications at a young age. In fact, the average expected lifespan of a person with type 1 diabetes is now the same as for a person without it.

Help your teen see that daily care helps them feel good in the moment. See if he or she can understand that more erratic blood sugars (because with the tools available today, no one with type 1 diabetes can avoid some erratic blood sugars) can lead to exhaustion, difficulty focusing, and other immediate physical maladies. That should be the focus for teens, not a fear of complications or death looming ahead of them.

You can do this with written and verbal information. Share with them when you read promising studies. Show them adults who have lived long and well with type 1. Make sure they know to just shake their heads when some lady in the market spouts off about her old aunt losing a leg. Help them know, in their hearts, that their future is bright.

While setting a positive tone, though, you'll also want your teen to know that sometimes it's okay to be sick of diabetes. Help teens learn not just how to voice that feeling, but to find ways to make themselves feel better when they do. Be it asking you to take over more of their care, or having a group of friends who truly get it and to whom they can vent (diabetes camp friends are great for this), or just knowing that sometimes in life we all need a (short) pity party, help them learn that they don't have to hide their negative

Check Your Own Tone

If you feel sorry for yourself as the parent of a child with diabetes or often send a message about how hard it is or how much you hate it, you'll need to find a way to work on your own outlook. Even if you think you're not saying it when your child is around, our teens pick up cues on what we think and how we feel. Find the good in it as well and model that for your child.

feelings. In fact, sharing them is the best thing they can do to move past them, or at least live with them. You may also want to talk to them, frankly, about what depression is and how it can impact many people with diabetes. Help them to understand the signs themselves, and see if they can become cognizant of what they might or might not be feeling. This is not a small task with teens. But sometimes even if they don't seem to be listening, they are indeed.

When Action Is Needed

If you do see signs of depression, the first action you'll want to take is to call your child's medical team and discuss your concerns. Ask them for guidance and support and, if possible, to set up an emergency appointment to meet with and assess your teen's state of mind. From there, you'll need to be sure you have good therapeutic care that works in harmony with the teen's diabetes medical team.

If you have that in place, the team should be able to help guide you, even to the point of whether your child needs hospitalization for depression. Remember: it is complicated and challenging to sort out what is depression, what is burnout, what is a combination, what can be helped slowly along with therapeutic care, and what needs drastic and immediate intervention. Having a team you trust onboard to help you and your teen with all this is paramount.

But what if you don't have a team onboard that you trust at the moment, and you fear for your child's safety?

> **Depression and Daily Care**
>
> A teen suffering from depression cannot handle daily diabetes care, and you'll need to take it all back on if you are not handling it already. Depression can leave people unable to brush their own teeth. Diabetes care must be handled by another person when a teen is depressed.

You'll want to protect your child, and if a hospital setting is the only way you feel you can do that, you'll need to do it.

In most cases, this is not needed. But what is needed are parents or other adults who are supportive, willing to learn, and ready to patiently help teens along as they gain their footing again and work toward a place where they can hold depression at bay.

Eating Disorders

When you think about how much food becomes the center of life with type 1 diabetes around, it's hard to imagine how children growing up with it *don't* develop eating issues. Thankfully, a vast majority do not. That said, teens with diabetes do face a higher chance of developing eating disorders than teens without diabetes. And usually, that disorder involves the omission of insulin. In fact, a study published in the prestigious *New England Journal of Medicine* found that 30 percent of adolescent females with type 1 diabetes had omitted insulin as a weight loss measure. No study is available on males and this topic, but it does seem to affect females more (as do all eating disorders).

So what happens in the mind? Start with the fact that diabetes is all about focusing on food. After all, children with diabetes grow up knowing the carb count of just about everything out there. They watch as their parents count every carb on their plate and stress over meal plans and food logbooks. They have to think every single time they eat. That can overflow into a feeling of wanting to control food rather than having food seemingly controlling them.

Add to that the intense pressure society

> **Boys and Eating Disorders**
>
> While it is less common, males can suffer from eating disorders. If you have a son with diabetes, read on and learn the symptoms, just in case.

puts on girls in particular to be thin and "beautiful." When teens realize that high blood sugars and omitted insulin can actually cause them to lose weight, the temptation can be extreme. The combination of succumbing to that temptation and developing eating disorders is what the general public calls "diabulimia." The medical term for it, however, is ED-DMT1, which looks at the eating disorder and the insulin omission as two distinct but interwoven situations.

A person does not have to be overweight to be susceptible to eating disorders and insulin omission for weight manipulation. In fact, teens who are underweight, overweight, and average weight have all suffered with this condition.

Usually, the eating issues develop first. You may notice teens changing their eating habits, eating way less or way more. You may find evidence of hoarding (such as wrappers in a drawer or food hidden in a bedroom). Of course, fluctuations in weight could be a sign as well. While you don't weigh your teen, you may notice clothing fitting in a different way or see them dress to hide how their clothing is fitting.

As for the insulin manipulation, signs of this include unexplained high blood sugars on a more frequent basis, insulin not needing to be refilled as often, and even, in extreme cases, DKA and hospital admission.

Here it is important to note that even that kind of sign can be overlooked. Parents, for the most part, don't want to believe their child could suffer like this and may be in denial. Teens can come up with "reasons" for their DKA or highs (pump malfunction, insulin got hot, forgot to check a couple of times), and parents can accept that. It is important to at least consider privately the possibility of omitted insulin if you see more frequent highs, a hospitalization, or a lack of insulin being used. It's better to consider it and be wrong than not consider it and have your child end up in a dangerous situation.

Treatment of and Complications from Eating Disorders

Besides the obvious immediate side effects such as sickness, exhaustion, inability to focus and function, and weight loss, eating disorders can wreak long-term havoc on a body. Even for the person without diabetes, this is true. But with diabetes, like most other things, it means even more danger. Long-time elevated blood sugars can indeed lead to complications. The problem is, telling a teen this will only backfire. Most teens who are struggling with eating issues, when told to stop so they don't cause complications, think this: "I'll be dead by then anyway. It's already too late." Threats of what may happen do not help.

Instead, you'll need to put your child and yourself in the hands of an expert who knows how to help a person recover from this situation. Your medical team should be able to help you with that, finding an eating disorder team that understands ED-DMT1 and can help your child work through it, and help you learn how to support the child in that goal. No doubt about it, success is more likely through a family effort.

There are inpatient facilities for this situation as well, but not in every state. If your child needs inpatient care, it may involve going to a facility somewhere not close to your home, which is a huge undertaking. The medical team can help you with that decision as well.

How does a parent avoid this in the first place? Some experts think eating disorders are born in the chemical balance of a person, much as depression and other emotional issues can be. But you can start early to try to not make food as big a deal. If children want to eat something, show them the answer can most always be "yes" (just with insulin along). Encourage them to just treat food as any other child would—something they enjoy when they want to and eat when they should.

Drug Abuse and Type 1 Diabetes

No parents want their children to experiment with drugs. The parent of the child with diabetes feels this even more so. That drug abuse is illegal, dangerous, and just wrong does not need to be pointed out.

Teens who abuse drugs tend to have a higher average blood sugar, poorer daily control, and more chance of a DKA situation or a dangerous low. And yet, the pressure, fear, worry, and stress of diabetes can lead a teen to seek out drug use as an escape. Once again, the irony is that the drug use only complicates the daily life with diabetes more.

Teens who experiment with drugs and have diabetes need to be taken seriously from the start. Since insulin can be a dangerous thing when it is misused, and drug use can impair the mind's ability to work well, any drug use is a danger. While some parents may shake off experimentation, parents of teens with diabetes need to take action immediately.

First of all, you need to consider the possibility of long-term struggles. Studies show that the younger a teen begins experimenting with drugs, the more chance there is of long-term addiction issues. Older teens, from 17 on, have less of a chance (but still have a chance). Then you need to consider that the body of a child with diabetes needs extra good care. Drug use works counter to that. Since the teen mind tends not to listen, your sharing this information might not help outwardly. But finding a way for the teen to consider this won't hurt.

If you discover your child has used an illegal drug (and that includes any prescription drugs they may "borrow" from home), contact his or her medical team immediately and get a plan of action in place. Counseling and intervention may be needed.

If your child ends up in a situation that requires rehab, you'll need to find a rehab that understands—and embraces—the unique challenges of drug abuse and diabetes. They do exist and are strongly recommended if you face this challenge.

But what about marijuana, now legal in two states and possibly to become legal in more? As this book is published, pot use is still against Federal laws. As a parent, you need to remind your child of that. Beyond that, smoking in itself is not a good idea with diabetes onboard. You'll want to talk to your child about why smoking can affect a person with diabetes more than others, and discuss how smoking pot has the same impact as cigarettes in that way.

Here is another thing for your teen to consider about pot use: it impairs your ability to make educated choices. Since a person with diabetes needs to always be thinking of things like insulin doses, blood sugars, and more, impairing the ability to think clearly can be not just a bad idea, but a truly dangerous idea. While perhaps teens without diabetes can ask a friend to drive them home or watch out for them, teens with diabetes usually cannot ask someone to watch their diabetes for them.

As more and more states move toward legalizing pot, this could be as important a subject as alcohol in coming years. As with alcohol, you should make sure your teen knows the facts and knows he or she can be honest with you even after making a decision you might not approve of. Safety first.

In the end, it is your job as a parent to intervene and protect your child when it comes to dangerous situations. Doing your best to educate and encourage good choices, and then keeping an eye out for signs of a bad situation will keep you ahead of things. Knowing what to do and doing it will help your teen move toward a better time.

And should it seem like a battle, remember this: in the end, teens *want* to feel good, both physically and emotionally. While they may give you pushback and battle you, when they turn the corner and feel good again, they'll thank you for doing your job as a parent.

CHAPTER FOURTEEN

Transitioning to Self-Care

All I had to do to remind myself of how not ready I knew my daughter was to begin to take over managing her diabetes care was glance into her bedroom. You know, the room with the mess of clothes on the floor, the pile of papers that might just be important for school, and the mishmash of pocketbooks, cell phone cords, and goodness knows what else strewn all over the place? No way, I'd think to myself, is she qualified or prepared to take on managing all that goes into diabetes care.

But I was wrong. Because here's the thing: like it or not, our goal as parents is to raise our kids and then ease them into taking responsibility in life for better or for worse. While in my head I felt there was no way my daughter could possibly be organized and responsible enough to manage diabetes, in my heart I knew, deep down, I had to help her do just that, for better or for worse.

I'll be honest: I had some ego wrapped up in all of this. For years and years, I'd been the rock star mom; the one who could juggle prescriptions with my eyes closed, convince the front desk worker to squeeze an endo appointment in where the chart showed there was no room for one, and make diabetes a seamless overlay in my daughter's life. I was needed. And it's hard to even think about letting that go. After all, we parents need to feel needed, don't we?

I might never have let it go were it not for my (always) wise daughter, who insisted the process begin, and did things to push it along when it sputtered. Today, while I still manage some of her diabetes needs, the majority of the job is hers.

As for that bedroom, it can still be a mess sometimes. But I've learned that in life, a messy room does not always fore-shadow the rest of a person's life. And sometimes, a kid might just have a messy room because that's not important. What is important, they rise up to and master.

Transitioning teens' diabetes care from your full supervision to something they handle on their own is not done with the snap of a finger. Rather, transitioning is a slow, steady, and hopefully well-thought-out process that can span years. In fact, your teen's medical team may already be moving toward that goal without your even realizing it.

Why is it important to transition? Put simply, we want to raise our children to be self-reliant and responsible adults who thrive. That, perhaps, is our most important goal as a parent: raising a child who becomes an adult who not only copes but does well in the world on their own.

If you think about it, you've become a "transition expert" over the years of parenting you've put in. For kids with diabetes and for all other kids as well, life is about transitioning to personal responsibility and freedom. You sit back and sip coffee while they work out a sharing issue at playgroup as a toddler, for the first time letting them figure that out themselves. You send them off to kindergarten, allowing them to learn to behave without you coaching them along. You help them adapt to grade school, keeping track of homework assignments for them and eventually showing them how to keep track themselves. You drop them off at sleepovers, trusting them for an evening and into the morning to do all they are supposed to do. As they grow, you leave it to them more and more to know where they are supposed to be and for how long. It's called slowly growing up.

With diabetes onboard, this is even more important. It's easy for a teen to keep feeling like a child—one who cannot plan or do things independently—if the complicated world of planning things with diabetes onboard has always been shielded from that teen. True, we do the shielding out of love: who wants to have a child realize the sometimes seemingly endless details that go into children's lives in general? But as they get older and clued in, the more we shield them, the more they may begin to think they are not capable of surviving on their own. Our instinct to protect and care for them can actually send a subliminal message to them that says they are not capable of caring for themselves. And this is not a good thing.

When Is the Time Right?

So how soon does a parent (and medical team) begin working toward transitioning care? Baby steps can be taken quite early. Things like having children look on as you log blood glucose numbers (or having them share an app you use to do just that, even if it's just to look on in interest) can happen from an early age. So can having them do things like draw the insulin up into the needle. Or change the lancet on their pricker (you do change it, right?). These little steps can happen all along the diabetes road.

But the true work toward transitioning should begin in the early teen years. This way, you and your teen's medical team can ease your child into understanding how to handle things, knowing what goes into it, and, most importantly, voicing what the teen is ready for and not ready for as he or she goes along. Some say your goal should be for teens to be completely self-reliant by the time they leave for college. Others feel that it's fine to still be managing things such as prescriptions and appointments at that point. That is up to you and your child. But one thing is for sure: by the time teens are 18, they should understand the ramifications of daily diabetes care and the details that go into being self-reliant in that way.

That's not to say all teens are equal in their readiness to take this on. Of course, we all mature at different speeds. While some kids seem ready to conquer all this on their own even before they are officially teens, others seem not ready even when they are well into their teens. So, is there a hard and fast rule about age? No,

> ### Some Things Are for the Long Term
>
> Some parents like to hold onto control of things, such as prescription refills and appointment management. This is fine for the time being, particularly if the child (or young adult) is still on your insurance. Some parents oversee the prescriptions for years into their child's adulthood. It's a way to say "I still care" once the child is out of the house.

but there are some guidelines. On the lower end of age, this is clear: even if your child seems ready to take things on without your oversight, don't go there yet. Young teens and preteens—even the most mature and responsible ones—need parental oversight even if they don't think they do. Handing over full diabetes care at a young age can lead to burnout, as well as to mistakes.

On the other end of that spectrum, by the time teens move toward legal driving age, they should be ready to begin taking steps toward some self-management. After all, college and the "real world" are only a couple of years away. If teens want to go off to college or out to work in the real world, they need to be ready to begin accepting bits and pieces of their care before they get to that point.

If your teen refuses all steps toward any independence, you'll want to discuss this with the teen's medical team and the team's social worker. If they feel your child is pushing back when he or she should be moving forward, you may want to consider counseling. But there can be reasons too: a teen who has suffered burnout or is moving toward it may need you to take over care, at least for a while. (Refer to chapter 12 for details.)

The Endo Appointment: Moving Toward Independence

Usually in the child's early teens your endo team will begin to lead the way in the process of learning to be independent, doing things like having your child attend half of the appointment without you in the room. This can be shocking—and sometimes upsetting—to a parent. What, you think, could your child possibly need to talk about or learn without you hearing it all? But the truth is, there are topics your teen needs to discuss with the medical team out of your earshot. And more than that, teens need to begin to develop confidence in their own ability to not only communicate with a doctor, but to advocate for themselves in a medical setting. In fact, this might be one of the most important skills your teen with diabetes learns over these years.

So here's the first step in how medical appointments work as your teen transitions from you, the parent: you need to set your own ego, fears, and notions aside and just let some of this begin to happen out of your earshot.

For the time being (and at least until your teen is 18), the medical team should call you into the room for at least part of the appointment. Some teams like to do the parent section first, to avoid having the parent come in and quiz everyone about what might have been discussed while the parent was out of the room. And remember, in the car on the way home or days down the road, do *not* ask your teen what was discussed while you were out of the room. That is the teen's information to keep private. And if a teen wants to discuss it with you, he or she will bring it up.

Even when you are in the room, this is the time to move toward letting your teen's voice be the first one heard. If your child has had T1D for a long time, you are probably used to steering the ship, and your teen probably is used to you doing so. But now, when asked a question, try to defer to your teen to respond. The medical team should help with this, encouraging the teen with eye contact and questions to help your teen express what he or she is thinking. Parents don't need to be mute; you are still an important part of this team. But they do need to speak less and listen more, allowing the teen to run the appointment.

It's on the Record

Remember, your medical team should be keeping a record of what goes on in appointments and sending you a follow-up note after each appointment. This is where you can still keep track. If your team is not doing this, request that they begin doing it now. But do have them send a copy to your child. Remember, your goal is for the teen to take ownership of all this.

This means some work for you to help your teen prepare before the appointment as well. You've probably always made a list of things you want to be sure to bring up and discuss at appointments. Before your next appointment, share this process with your teen and encourage him or her to make a list, too. If teens have a day planner, have them jot down thoughts on a page in there. (Also tell them you start the list a week before and keep adding to it, because no one can think of everything in one shot. You *do* do that, right? Well, if you don't you can start now along with your teen). If they don't use a day planner, have them use the notes app on their smartphone, because you know they have those! Give them some prompts the first time ("I notice you don't like checking two hours after lunch. Do you want to talk about that at the appointment?") Let them know, too, that there will absolutely be a time they can ask questions out of your earshot, and that they can keep their list of questions and concerns to be brought up at the appointment private as well if they would like. Remind them the first few times to bring their list and to have it in front of them at the appointment. Tell them it's fine to check off each item to be sure they covered it. Let them know that many times you have left an appointment wishing you'd not forgotten something. This will help them learn how to manage not just medical appointments, but all appointments and meetings in their lives.

Compromise and Letting Some Things Go

As your teen moves toward independence (along with the help of their medical team), you the parent may find you have to let some things go. Because here's a tip: your idea of how to manage T1D on a daily basis may differ somewhat from your teen's. And really, so long as a teen's medical team is onboard, whatever he or she decides has to be okay with you.

This is not at all easy for parents. For instance, teens often balk at frequent blood glucose checking. While you may have done ten or more checks a day when they were younger, they may not want to commit to that anymore. So here's the scenario: your teen tells the medical team that he or she would like to check less during the day and night. The teen has valid reasons (and for most medical teams, "I'm sick of it," can be a valid reason). Teen and doctor come up with a modified checking plan that both agree to, but that is far from what you as a parent prefer.

What are you to do? You have to compromise. First, it is okay to express your feelings at the appointment and with your teen and the doctors in the room. Saying something like "I know you don't want to check two hours after lunch but that scares me" is fine. Then, you have to listen. And if the medical team is onboard with the changes, you need to accept and adapt. Remember, your teen's medical team is not going to be onboard with anything that is unsafe or counterproductive. This will feel very much like a leap of faith for you as a parent because really, it is. But it is a leap you need to take in order to help your teen move toward independence.

Here's another thing you may need to let go of: constant supervision of every single meter check and insulin dose. Of course there are situations that are exceptions to this. For instance, teens who have recently fallen into danger or trouble with their diabetes care may be in need of your constant oversight. If this is the case, you'll work with their medical team for them to understand this (more in chapters 11 and 12). But in the case of the average teen, it may be time for you to just oversee averages, trends, and insulin changes.

Teens get sick of hearing from you every single time they bolus or check or correct or change out a site. Here's the thing parents need to realize: teens are stuck thinking about this all the time. Having the added layer of hearing you talk about it all the time can drive them crazy. As long as they grow, as long as you know they are trying and not in any kind of trouble, you may need to back off from the constant diabetes interaction.

Again, this can come via the medical team and your teen. You should feel free to express your fears at an appointment ("I'm afraid he/she will just stop checking if I am not watching over constantly" is something you might say). Just be prepared to hear that you need to give the teen a chance, in fact, some checks might be forgotten, and it's still going to be okay.

Another compromise may come in how teens administer their insulin and check their blood sugar. Often, teens crave change just for the sake of change. This might mean a teen who has been on an insulin pump for years and years suddenly wants to switch to shots. Parents who are pump advocates can cringe at this. But in the end, you need to allow your teen to use the system he or she wants to use for insulin administration. Again, the teen's medical team would be involved in this decision. As a parent, you can again express your fears, but in the end you need to go along with the decision that your teen and the medical team make.

The same goes for CGM use. If you really want your teen to use one but he or she flat-out refuses, you need to respect that. But ask for compromise here for you. Might your teen be willing to wear a CGM one week out of each month? See if you can win teens over to your way a tiny bit. And if you cannot, again, it's their body and their decision at this point. You want to raise them to think things through, come up with a decision, and then advocate for it. If that means something you want isn't going to happen, you may just have to settle for that, for the sake of your teen.

Remember, for now, diabetes is a lifetime thing. Teens are going to have many years ahead of them to consider new devices and try new plans. Let them work their way to such things on their own time.

The biggest compromise of all may be what an acceptable A1C is. Parents are particularly bogged down with A1C results (some call them the SATs of diabetes). You probably worked hard to keep that number down for years and years. The teen years, with hormones, growth spurts, and free will, can be a time of challenge for A1Cs. Listen to your teen's medical team and what numbers they feel are okay. And if it is higher, don't freak out. Instead, help your teen work positively toward a lower A1C. And accept that it might take time.

Time for an Adult Endo?

The fact is, most pediatric endocrinology teams will continue to see patients through their college years and sometimes even longer. Some teens and young adults with diabetes like that: they feel comfortable with their same practice and are not ready to make a change. If they are happy and feel well cared for and understood, there is no reason to make a change.

But sometimes, teens grow to face adult issues and problems and challenges that some pediatric groups don't have as deep an understanding of as adult practices do. If your teen feels this is the case (or you do), it's time to consider an adult practice.

Some pediatric practices will tell you that adult endos don't have the same connection or compassion that pediatrics do. This is not always the case. If you shop around and let your teen talk to a few, he or she is bound to find one with whom they connect. Sometimes, the shift to an adult endo is just what the teen needs to get things back on track.

Most adult endos don't take patients until they are 18, but if your teen shops around and asks, explaining they feel a need to transition to adult care, some adult endos will take them on.

Remember, this is a time when you can help teens with research and with helping them think about what they are looking for in a practice, but at the end of the day, they will have to do most of the communicating. After all, that's what adults do. Still, with your teen's permission, adult endos will share information and have discussions with you as well. They will, however, expect their patients to be the leaders, not the parents.

Parental Involvement Long Term—How to Stay in the Loop

Once the parent of a child with diabetes, always the parent of a child with diabetes. It does not matter if your child is 14 or 40, or even older, it is impossible to turn off your parental instinct and care. And really, you don't have to.

Because forever and ever, you are a teen's parent. And there are ways to stay looped in (sustaining inter-dependence), not just as teens move toward independence, but once they get there. Some ideas include:

- Driving to and from their medical appointments with them (if they live in the same general area as you). True, once they are adults you won't go into the doctor's office with them. But often, the ride to and from the appointment is the longest time people with diabetes spend thinking about their diabetes. You being there to talk (or not talk) or listen can be a huge benefit to your child, and can keep you in the loop.
- Offering to help manage prescriptions. Even from a long distance, you can do this for your child for as long as you want to and the child wants to. Fighting with insurance can be lousy, and most parents of kids who grow up with diabetes have become masters. Taking this burden off your adult child's shoulders can help remind him or her

that you do care, and make you feel like you are still helping.

- Leave the door open to them sharing logbooks with you and asking for information. Let them know that you would always be happy to look for trends and things in their numbers, and that they can send them to you any time. And if they do, don't judge, just help.

- Stay active in advocacy and fundraising. Even if your child moves on from it, do all you can to help work toward better treatments and a cure. This will remind them, daily, that you still care. And it will keep you in the loop about what is going on with research and daily care.

In the end, you want children to move on toward a life and care plan that they own. But you can let them know you are forever and always their parent. When they need you, you stand ready.

CHAPTER FIFTEEN

Advocacy and the Teen with Diabetes

I didn't really think about it until it was actually happening. I mean, I knew my teen daughter with diabetes was going to be part of the 2008 Democratic National Convention. I was witness to Senator Ted Kennedy asking her to be part of his tribute video, and I was at historic Hyannis Port when famed filmmaker Ken Burns shot my daughter's part. (Her teen takeaway from that amazing day: "Wow. I wish his hair and makeup people could fix me up every day." Kids.) But the night the tribute ran, as my family and I sat in our living room watching, I got chills like I'd never had before.

Not only was it crazy exciting to see my child become part of history (and she is—to this day she is part of the display at *the Kennedy Library in Boston), but it blew me away to see what she instinctively did with it. Because my daughter, the well-trained advocate, knew how to phrase her wording so that the message deep in her heart—for awareness about type 1 diabetes and her organization of choice, JDRF—would have to be left in. I looked over at her when it wrapped and said, "Wow. Not only was that great, you nailed your message while still saluting the senator."*

She winked at me. "I had a plan, Mom. I had a plan."

The years of advocacy we experienced as a family were not always simple. Over the years, I had to be careful to always remember that Lauren was a teen first and an advocate for diabetes research second. While there were times I wanted her to absolutely say "yes" to anything anyone asked her to do (she was so good at it and it was really amazing to see her learn from the experiences; I wanted a cure.), I had to remember to let her be the driver. (Okay, and a few times when I just knew she had to say yes I might have bribed her.)

Advocacy gave her so much back, though. Few are surprised that Lauren chose to major in government and communications in college in Washington, D.C., and hopes to pursue a career in public service. You'll read her thoughts on her experience at the end of this chapter.

As the mom of an advocate and as an advocate myself, I hope this chapter helps you and your teen consider getting involved, but doing it in a way that does not negatively affect your child.

Advocates can have some wonderful experiences. You might not always end up having Ken Burns's team spiffing you up, but you can end up feeling like you've helped change the world. It can also give a teen a feeling of power in a world that sometimes tries to make teens feel powerless. When blood sugars won't cooperate, they can still make their voices heard. And even bored teens have a hard time not loving that feeling.

Deciding to become an advocate is an important decision that teens and their parents need to think over carefully. If you've never stepped up before and are considering it now, you and your teen will want to talk over all sides of it. And if you've long been a parent advocate along with a child who did a lot in preteen years, it's important you visit the topic with your teen now. Not all teens want to be active and visible in the diabetes advocacy world. Even if your teen loved it as a smaller child, you'll want to gauge his or her interest in it and feelings about it at this time, to be sure you are not pushing the teen into a place or a movement he or she just doesn't want to be part of right now.

First, let's answer a simple question: exactly what is advocacy? The dictionary defines it this way: "to speak or write in favor of; support or urge by argument; recommend publicly: he advocated higher salaries for teachers." To put that simply: advocacy in the diabetes world means being willing to speak out, write about, ask friends to listen about, and work toward making things happen about understanding what diabetes is, why funding for a cure is needed, and how people can help.

How do you know if advocacy is right for your teen? Folks commonly think that the more outgoing, leader-type teen is the type to want to be a part of all this. While it's true this type of personality may lend itself well to advocacy roles, parents of quieter children are often surprised to see them come alive at an advocacy event, speaking up about things they barely mention at home, embracing the chance to make a difference for themselves and for others. What that means is you really cannot judge a book by its cover when it comes to advocacy and teens.

It's a good idea to at least expose teens to programs and ways they can make a difference. Even teens who say "no way" with little discussion should be given a glimpse of what is out there for them because the benefits can become meaningful to them over time.

Advocacy Benefits

Of course you want your teen to want to become an advocate for the purest of reasons: to help the world and to help move us toward better living with diabetes and a cure. But it's okay to realize and accept (and share) that there are many more benefits teens can glean from being advocates. Some are tangible (and might motivate them more); others are less tangible (but will be meaningful to them in the long run). Help your teen understand what advocacy can bring to him or her while helping others.

The tangible benefits are simple and somewhat basic. First off, most teens today need to complete some kind of community service to graduate from high school. Taking part in diabetes advocacy programs can be a way for them to do that while at the same time learning more about the advocacy/cure/government landscape and diabetes. Have teens find out what their required hours are (and remember, if they are interested in something like the National Honor Society, there are probably additional hour requirements— make sure they ask early so they can plan ahead for this). Then, reach out to a diabetes organization and ask how your teen can help. There are suggestions of places and programs later in this chapter.

Advocacy programs and experiences can also lend themselves well to school homework, projects, and extra credit. For instance, if your teen decides that he or she wants to meet with an elected official, the teen will need to study up on who the elected official is, how that official's position works, and how the official can help the diabetes world. All that is truly educational and can be used in a school paper or project. Sometimes, when a project is assigned, parents have an opening to suggest an advocacy program to the teen as part of the project.

If a teen agrees to speak at an event or write a letter as part of a program, encourage the teen to see if his or her English teacher or writing teacher will consider making it an assignment or at least an extra credit project. Learning to speak and to write in a way that wins over support is a challenging and important skill to build. If a teacher will support that effort, your child could not only learn more but earn some extra credit or find a way to make an assignment more interesting.

Team Effort

Often, high school sports teams are required to do community service hours as a group. While some teens cringe at the idea of asking their teams to do something "for them," it's a great idea for teams to rally behind a player. Have teens talk to their coaches about how the team can advocate alongside them.

And of course there is the all-consuming college application.

With college acceptance as competitive as it is today, the more teens can add to their applications, the better. And here's where your teen "lucks out" (although using the word "luck" with diabetes doesn't quite feel right): there is a sea of teens trying to fit some kind of community service into their high school time just to put it on an application. College selection folks are adept at sniffing out the many teens that just do it to check off the box. Your teen is absolutely doing it for a true, honest, personal, and important reason. That will shine through on an application, as well as give the teen something to write a great essay about. It might possibly give the teen a nice recommendation letter as well. While elected official letters are often frowned upon by college admissions offices (so many parents just call in favors for them, and again, admissions officers know how to sniff those out), if your child meets with an elected official, advocates, and makes a difference, that just might earn the right for a meaningful letter that would outshine those basic ones other kids might have.

It's Not Required in Life

It's important to say this and remind ourselves of it all the time: just because teens have type 1 diabetes does not mean they have an obligation to advocate for a cure or help the diabetes world. If it's up their alley and they are interested, that's great. But they did not sign on for this disease or to be a "face of it." So in the end, respect their decision either way.

It's important here to discuss the college application and similar efforts. Many teens balk at the idea of "using" diabetes on their college applications or "playing the diabetes card." This is probably because you've raised them right and taught them that they are people first and people with diabetes second, and that diabetes should not differentiate them from the many other teens in the world. But we all know: it does. Your teen has had to be brave, smart, determined, patient, balanced, and more just to live his or her life. And that means something to admissions officers. Encourage teens with diabetes to embrace this fact. Remind them that you're not telling them to whine about diabetes or to brag about it, but merely to share what diabetes has done to help shape them as people. They've paid a big price in life thanks to diabetes. They deserve to get something back from it, and if their hard work in living this life and in advocacy gives them that, more power to them. Remember, this may take some convincing from you or their guidance counselor. But do work at convincing them.

Another benefit from advocacy work can actually be health and well-being, both emotional and physical. First and foremost, advocacy can help connect a teen to other teens with diabetes. We know as parents that there is power in numbers, specifically in numbers of people we connect with who understand this world we live in. Chances are your teen does not know many other teens in his or her school with diabetes, and if there are some, they might not share enough to be friends. In the advocacy world, they'll work with, get to know, and usually bond with others who get it and who can talk to them confidentially and compassionately about what they are all going through.

So, too, can advocacy help teens see down the road. Hearing adults or seniors talk about how they've thrived despite diabetes can be powerful for a teen (even if they don't admit it to you). Meeting a celebrity with diabetes can have an impact as well. And having to learn about what kind of research is out there, what breakthroughs have come, and what might happen down the road helps them have hope for a brighter future.

Most of all, a teen who may be feeling beaten down about life with diabetes can find some power and progress via advocacy. Let's say your teen agrees to speak at a walk to cure diabetes rally. The teen might be a bit annoyed at having to do the work and actually

ADVOCACY FROM A TEEN PERSPECTIVE

I became a diabetes advocate probably before I even knew what the word "advocate" meant. I can remember being about seven years old and speaking at a business event about the JDRF Walk to Cure Diabetes. My mother was always sure to let me tell my own story, not one she wanted me to tell, and I did just that on that day.

After I spoke, a man came up to me and told me he was going to have his company donate a LOT of money to the walk because of what I said. That stuck with me: my words, my story, and my being willing to speak up could help change the world. It was an awesome feeling.

By the time I was a teen, I had a lot of advocacy experience. I have to say that even though I was struggling with burnout and all, being an advocate helped me so much in those years because even on my hardest, worst days I was still doing something positive.

I would suggest all teens consider doing some advocacy work in the diabetes world. First of all, it does give you that feeling of making a difference. Second, you can meet some really amazing people and friends through it. Third, it's an educational experience that really will help you in your future.

I have been able to be part of lobbying for bills to be passed. I have spoken before Congress twice. I even got to speak at the 2008 Democratic National Convention in the tribute to Senator Ted Kennedy. I have been on CNN *Live* a few times, on *NOVA*, on *Good Morning America*, and in too many other media things to count. I was chosen to be Chairkid of JDRF's Children's Congress, one of the most important positions a kid with diabetes can hold. In many ways, I have been so lucky.

While not everyone will have the same experience I will have, everyone can make a difference. Figure out what you are interested in: speaking, or volunteering to help other kids with diabetes, or fund-raising, or a combination. Then find a way to make it happen.

One piece of advice I would give parents is this: Don't force your child to do this. Get children to try some, and hopefully they'll want to do more. My mother always gave me an option when I was asked to do things to say no (and quite a few times I did say no). While my mom and I shared a lot of the advocacy experiences, in the end, it was mine to do or not do. That, I think, is important to remember.

I have had diabetes going on 16 years now. It has given me a lot of scary things—like lows and highs and shots and finger pricks. But it also helped me find my future. I am majoring in political communications at George Mason University now. (I'll graduate in 2013!) I love my career choice. Would I have found it without diabetes? We will never know. But I do know that I found it with diabetes. It's nice to make a difference, and it's exciting to be a part of change. All teens should try it.

Lauren Stanford

missing time online or with friends to go, but here's what happens right when the teen is done: he or she is surrounded by folks expressing thanks, telling the teen that *he* or *she* is a role model to a small child, and by folks waiting to shake hands and praising the teen for making a difference. It's not insulin, but that kind of feeling can be a powerful "medicine," too.

Awards and Scholarships: They're Out There

There's nothing wrong with getting to know the awards and scholarships that might be out there for the teen diabetes advocate. Again, teens with diabetes pay a high price each and every day. Winning a scholarship or award for going above and beyond in advocacy is a nice balance to all that sacrifice. Some awards to research (you can easily Google each of them) include:

- **The Prudential Spirit of Community Award.** Two are awarded annually in each state, and from among those, ten national winners are chosen. Winners are students who have shown exemplary dedication to a program or a project that makes a difference in lives. More than a few teens with diabetes have won this honor, including a national winner in 2005.

- **DoSomething.org.** Do something is a program created by Hollywood celebrities to encourage teens and young adults to make a difference in the world. Joining Do Something guides teens through advocacy programs (even offering boot camps on how to be an advocate) and grants to help teens build programs. They offer scholarships and awards regularly to teens who build and promote their work through them. Even teens who partner with groups like JDRF and ADA can still use this group to better their efforts, and of course to win grants and scholarships.

- **The Diabetes Scholars Program.** This program has grown to the point of now offering dozens and dozens of scholarships annually for teens heading off to college who also have diabetes. Grades, leadership, and personal story are all considered.
- **JDRF Scholarships.** Debuted in 2012, JDRF now offers college scholarships for teens in such categories as advocacy, interest in government, and interest in science and the medical field. The administration of the scholar ships is managed via the Diabetes Scholars program.
- **Best Buy Scholarships.** Based more on community service than financial need, these scholarships are awarded to hundreds of teens across America each year.

You may also want to check with your teen's guidance office for any local scholarships that may be relevant to your teen's advocacy work. And don't forget to ask your child's college financial aid office once he or she selects a college. Many colleges offer scholarships to students with type 1. George Mason University in Fairfax, Virginia, for instance, offers a competitive scholarship for just that.

Advocacy Programs to Consider

You don't have to join up with an organization to advocate. Teens and their families can certainly do it on their own by writing letters to their elected officials or offering to speak at their local Rotary clubs or the like. But there are so many great programs that have been built up, it makes sense to join up with one of them (or more than one of them). First, there is power in numbers. Second, you don't need to re-create the wheel and instead can use your teen's passion and hard work to move things forward even more. And third, your teen will become part of a team and a community, the value of which we've discussed here.

How to choose? It's a personal decision, and one you can make for your teen, or better yet, involve your teen in. You will want to do some research to make sure whatever organization you partner with supports the same goals you do and uses their donations and money wisely. You may also want to ask around to see if other families with diabetes onboard do advocacy work and can share their experiences with you. In the end, the decision is yours. Here are some programs geared at teens with diabetes you may want to consider.

- **JDRF's Children's Congress.** Held every other year in early summer in Washington, D.C., Children's Congress (CC) brings 140 kids with diabetes ranging in ages 4 to 17 to Capitol Hill to lobby for support of research for a cure for diabetes. **Cool factor:** Children's Congress was created by a kid named Tommy Solo from Massachusetts. Tommy's mom and godmother were very involved in diabetes advocacy on Capitol Hill. One day Tommy said to them, "Much of this is about us kids. So why aren't we the ones speaking out?" From that came Children's Congress, one of the most visible advocacy events in the diabetes world. **Details:** Applications go online in August of the year before CC (and it happens in odd years, so for, say, the 2015 Children's Congress, you'd look for the application in August of 2014). A selected delegate and one guardian are flown to D.C. for two to three days of events that include meetings with celebrities, meetings with your elected officials, and attending a congressional hearing on diabetes. All expenses are paid. **The hard part:** Literally thousands of children apply, and only 150 are selected, so it's not easy to get to go. But trying is fun, too. All teens interested in advocacy should apply.

- **The JDRF Promise to Remember Me Campaign.** Taking place in even-numbered years, this program puts teens (and people of all ages with type 1 diabetes) in front of their senators and congressional representatives at meetings in the home district. **Cool factor:** There is no application process, and everyone is welcome to take part. Often, district office meetings are more intimate and longer than any meetings in D.C., giving teens more time to tell their stories and get to know their elected officials. **Details:** By signing up to be a JDRF advocate, your teen will be updated about Promise meetings coming up. Usually, a volunteer leader sets up a meeting and reaches out to anyone who has shown interest in the representative's district or in the case of a senator, the state. It's a chance to meet other teens and families with diabetes, since usually a good-sized group attends. **The hard part:** Often the meetings are during the school day and require a kid to miss some school time. But they are educational. Have teens discuss their reason for missing class with teachers ahead of time and they may cooperate more.

- **Friends for Life Conference.** Held every July in Orlando (get past that—you won't mind the heat when you are there), this conference brings together more than 3,000 people who either have diabetes or care about someone who does. Created and run by the folks at childrenwith diabetes.com, it is said to be the largest gathering of its type in the world.

Cool factor: Teens get so much out of this event, with programs just for them such as driving tips with NASCAR star (and person with type 1) Charlie Kimball, tips on living with diabetes from celebrities like Crystal Bowersox, a day on their own (with chaperones and not their parents) at Disney, and even their own semiformal dinner dance. Watching the teens bond and become role models to younger kids at FFL is one of the most amazing parts of the program. Details: FFL offers something for everyone in the family, from educational sessions to a giant exhibit hall to world-famous speakers to down time when you just bond. Registration is up all year at the web site, and scholarships are available for the financially challenged. The hard part: It's Orlando. And it's July. But once you get there, you realize it's not hard at all since most of the event is indoors, and even when you are outdoors you are chilling with new friends.

- **The American Diabetes Association Call to Congress.** Every two years, the ADA brings a large group of folks with diabetes—both type 1 and type 2—to Washington, D.C., to call on Congress to ask for support of programs for people with diabetes and research for a cure. **Cool factor:** You get to meet and work with a large group of folks with diabetes of all ages. **Details:** Applications are online in the summer every other year, and you can apply and attend more than once. The event includes education, events, and visits to Capitol Hill.

- **The American Diabetes Association's National Youth Advocate program.** Each year, the ADA chooses one teen to represent all youth with diabetes in the nation. **Cool factor:** This leader travels the country and makes appearances, as well as writes a widely publicized blog. **Details:** Applications can be found at the ADA web site.

- **The Diabetes Research Institute's Diabetes Diplomats Program.** Any teen (or any person at all for that matter) can sign up and swing into action with this program that looks to support teens in holding fund-raising and educational events in their own communities. **Cool factor:** You can link in other areas of your life with this program, such as your student council or sports team or whatever you'd like. **Details:** Sign up at diabetesresearch.org/diabetesdiplomats.

Of course, there are other ways. Ask your endo team about any local support programs that may need your teen's help, or encourage your teen to start a group. Your local diabetes camp may use teens as advocates and certainly has a leadership training program they can take part in. Most groups such as JDRF and ADA and camps often need teens to do things like speak at events, meet with business leaders, or write letters asking for support. The best thing you can do is just call and ask.

But here's another idea: if you can, get your teen to call and ask. Nothing shows potential to these groups more than teens who will reach out on their own. But even if your teen won't, do it for him or her and help get the ball rolling. The end may just justify the means.

When to Take a Break

It's called the "poster child syndrome," and it can be very real. Particularly in cases with children who have been in the spotlight since they were young, advocacy can become a burden, something they resent or feel guilty about. It's vital that you keep an open dialogue with your teen (and your younger child) about any advocacy they do. When you are approached with an offer for your teen to do something like appear on television or speak at a gala or meet with someone to talk about diabetes, never, ever say yes without discussing it with the teen first.

Even if you really want your teen to do something, have the discussion. For teens, it's their diabetes, their face, their voice, and in the end, their decision about how to use that, to share it, or not to share it.

That said, there are times you can try to convince them to do something they might be on the fence about. For instance, let's say your teen was invited to take part in a public event on diabetes in which he or she would speak alongside a famed senator. Or a star athlete. You know that meeting and getting to know this person is going to benefit your teen in many ways (networking, knowing someone who has succeeded with diabetes onboard). It's okay to push your teen toward attending by pointing out the cool factor involved and the potential for great things to happen.

> **Role Models Struggle, Too**
>
> It's important to let your teen advocate know early on that even superstars in the diabetes world have rough patches. Find some examples of celebrities or well-known advocates talking about struggle and share it with teens.

But what if, even for invites that just seem amazing to you, your teen says no? Then no it must be. Because sometimes, a person just needs a break from all of this.

Teens pushed to be "poster children" can often rebel via their daily care. And if they are struggling with something like burnout, they may be too afraid to admit it, for fear of not just letting you down but also letting down all those people who have come to see them as a role model.

It can also become overwhelming for teens who are facing tons of homework, lots of AP classes, sports practice, and a part-time job to even wrap their heads around doing advocacy work. While it is true that we want to do all we can, always tell teens that it's their time and their life. And never forget: they never get even a moment off from their diabetes care. If they need time off from advocacy, so be it. You've shown them this world, and chances are, even if they take a break, eventually they will come back to it.

Because once you've given them the gift of understanding the power of their voice, they'll have that forever. Even after diabetes is cured.

CHAPTER SIXTEEN

Letting Them Go

It's not just parents of kids with diabetes who have trouble letting their kids go. I remember dropping my first child (who does not have T1D) off at college in New York City. I could barely imagine her ordering a new printer cartridge for her printer on her own, much less navigating life in a big city. But it was time, and we did it. With my daughter with diabetes, there was so much more at stake. Had I raised her to know what was right and wrong with diabetes aboard? Would she be sure to keep juice boxes and glucose tabs in supply? (Although as she pointed out when I dropped her off, I'd left her with enough supplies so that if every person in Washington, D.C., with diabetes were to visit her and need something at the same time, they'd all *be covered.) Would she remember to charge her cell phone in case she needed to call for help? Would she be fine without me?*

I am happy to report it all turned out well, with both girls. What I learned as I went along was this: we need to let them lead the way. Trust me, in most cases, our kids are ready to go off on their own, even if we think (or know, as it feels to us) they might not be quite there.

The summer before my daughter went off to school, we met with her adult endo. The two of them talked over some plans, and I barely said a word. When they were done, her doctor looked at me smiled and said this: "Mom, your girl is ready to fly."

He was right, of course. And the day I dropped her off, five hundred miles from our home, to begin her life on her own, I asked her just one thing: please, please let me know each morning that you woke up.

The next day, first thing, I heard my cell phone buzz. I picked it up and found a text from my daughter with diabetes.

"Good morning, Mom. I'm not dead!"

The humor she learned well. I smiled and hoped she'd learned the rest of it just as completely.

Of course we parents know the entire teen years' experience is a march toward independence. But when the time comes that you can see it on the horizon, we often feel surprised, shocked, and just plain not ready. But ready we must be: our job is not to raise lovely companions who remain by our side for eternity. Rather, our job as parents is to raise kind, positive, independent souls who go out in the world and contribute to it. It's no exaggeration to say that parenting well is among the most selfless acts around. We want them forever, but we've raised them up to send them out there in the world away from us.

This is why all the steps discussed in this book are vital. From the early teen years until they are adults (and beyond), the parents' role is to educate, support, and then, perhaps hardest of all, let go. To do this with a teen with T1D is, like anything else in this life with diabetes, a multi-layered challenge. Working toward it, as hard as it may feel, can bring the best reward of all: seeing your grown child thriving, happy and successful, out in his or her very own world.

Independence: It's Never Too Early to Get Ready

Let's say your teen is at that point of filling out college applications or thinking of applying for a technical apprenticeship or planning to be a ski bum or whatever that next step is in the teen's chosen life. While teens may only talk about which school or which trade or which mountain to make their own, you can be sure diabetes is weighing heavily on their minds. They own their diabetes, and you can be sure they're considering how on earth they are going to manage it away from the home they've known all their lives.

How can you help them see they can manage this? By doing what you hopefully have been doing: letting them experience freedom and independence in doses. Sleepovers, school trips, ski weekends with a friend's family, an overnight to an amusement park without you; whatever it is you let them do, they are all baby steps toward the big step of full independence.

What can a parent do to help teens move toward this step? Here are a few suggestions:

- **Begin looping them in on things like prescription and appointment management.** No, they do not have to do it on their own (and some parents, for logistical reasons, choose to keep managing these things through the college years or the first few years children are out on their own particularly if they are still on the family insurance). But they do need to begin to not only know what is going on, but how to handle it all. Show your teen how you manage prescriptions. (Do you use a calendar reminder? Do you automatically call in prescriptions when a certain amount is used? They need to learn all this.) Then, walk them through the process. Here's another idea: next time you have to make a phone call and fight for some coverage, have your teen listen in on another line. Not only will they see what you've been doing for them, they'll see that they don't always have to take the first answer they get as final. And when you keep a positive voice but still get your way, they'll learn from that, too. (Because you do that, right?) It's okay for them to see how a benefit card or any other insurance co-pays work, too. This can help them understand why securing a job and career with solid insurance is an important goal for them in life. As for appointment management, they'll need to know (and have written down) what appointments they need and when. While you can still help make them, they'll need to study their work and school schedules to help find the dates that work best, and then work with the doctor's office to coordinate an appointment time. As parents know, this is not easy. But showing them early on will help them learn to plan ahead for such things. Particularly if they are going to go far from home and keep the same medical team for a few years, they are going to have to learn to think ahead on such things.

- **Let them have their own time with their doctors.** If they are under 18 you can still be in there as much as you want, but encourage them, from as early an age as you can, to take some private time with their team to talk about what they wish. As they move toward heading off, the majority of time should actually be without you in there. Hopefully, they'll learn that sharing most with you is a positive thing, too. But let them figure that out. Feeling comfortable and confident sharing with a medical team is a good skill for teens to hone. They won't be able to truly hone it with you in the room.

- **Practice "passive communication."** There are parents of 40-year-olds with T1D who still discuss blood glucose trends with their children. This is all good and fine—after all, few are as expert in your child's diabetes as you are. But this usually comes from a choice made completely by the adult with diabetes, not by parents demanding to know what is going on. Most parents would like to end up in a place where their adult child still shares with them and asks their input and advice. How to get there? First, by not complaining if that is not where you get. Second, by finding ways early on to share and communicate in a passive way. We discussed earlier in this book about tools to share blood sugars that may help. Try to find a way, as you move toward college and life out there, for your teen to be willing to share information and for you to be willing to be quiet about it most of the time. This kind of backup support can lead to good sharing down the road, when young adults may feel they need it.

- **Work on *you*.** It's hard realizing our full-time job of raising them is about to shift to part-time, but we must let go with grace. Usually, the teens are way more ready that the parents for this step. You need to take time to think it all over. What are you afraid of? What are you excited about? What are you feeling guilty about? Talk to the parents of teens who have gone off to college or other places, and share with them your thoughts. And listen. You are going to hear how it all works out. Remember, the best parent is the selfless parent, and you are about to come to the time in the life of your teen when you have to be selfless, brave, and intuitive, and let teens go. If you find you are feeling overly scared or worried, you may want to check in with your doctor or counselor to work things out personally ahead of time. Don't let your own angst rob your child of this exciting next step in life.

College 101

If your child with diabetes is on the college track, you are probably worrying about frat parties, late nights, cafeteria food, and more. But know this: millions of teens with diabetes have gone to college. And rocked it.

> ### It's Not *Your* College Experience
>
> Remember, even if you are paying, this is not your college experience. It is your child's. Resist the urge to e-mail professors or go to the health office for the child. Teens who are not ready to do that on their own are not ready to go off to college on their own. If you let teens know it's their time to do these things, they usually will.

For any student, the transition from high school to college is a challenge. Even if students do not go away to school, they often face the same challenges as they take on the additional responsibilities of a full-time job, an apartment, and balancing a personal budget. It is often the first time young adults have the opportunity to make decisions without the supervision of their parents. For a typical college student this includes sleeping habits, homework, attending class, even keeping one's room clean. Those with diabetes are also expanding and navigating their increasing ability to make decisions regarding the care and management of their disease.

I have worked in higher education since 2003 at both public and private institutions in a variety of areas, such as orientation activities, disability services, academic advising, and career development. I have also had type 1 diabetes since 2002. As you can tell, I was diagnosed with type 1 diabetes in college, and it significantly changed my college experience. Learning about the processes of adult development and the structural and theoretical frameworks of the college environment after my diagnosis helped me better understand how the college experience can help people with diabetes and how parents can prepare their children to succeed in college and as adults with diabetes.

The typical college years of ages 18 to 22 is a time period of great intellectual, social, and emotional development. In recognition of that, colleges are structurally set up and plan activities to help encourage the development of the students. Intellectually, young adults are moving from individualistic concrete thinkers to understanding where their choices fit in relation to others. Young adults with diabetes may want their parents to solve the problems they encounter during college, including everything from remembering supply refills to roommate issues, but the college will encourage students to learn how to solve their problems on their own. The built-in support system makes college the best time for parents to take a step back and let their children learn on their own.

Students are navigating where they fit in the college environment, and diabetes will play a role as they navigate relationships with roommates, faculty, staff, and administrators, and in different situations including everything from internships to social events. For better or worse, diabetes provides the challenges and eventually the skills a young adult needs to be successful in life.

There are many organizations that do an excellent job of advocating for children with type 1 diabetes as they proceed through elementary and secondary school, making sure they receive the services that are needed and, in fact, required by law for them to receive equal and appropriate education. Because higher education is a privilege and not a legal requirement, the schools are not required to offer accommodations for students with diabetes or any other disability, unless the student chooses to self-disclose. As students develop their identities, those with diabetes are also facing the important decision to become advocates for their own health.

From a practical standpoint, college students with diabetes may request and be entitled to several different accommodations that will help them be successful in college. Students with diabetes are protected by the Americans with Disabilities Act and Section 504 of the Rehabilitation Act of 1973. It can be difficult to acknowledge diabetes as a disability. However, the law is clear, and people with diabetes are entitled to the protection. This protection is also not retroactive, so it is better to have accommodations on file and never use them than to end up in a situation where you wish there had been protection. Accommodations are not special privileges, but just ensure that the student receives the same educational opportunities as students without diabetes.

There is a variety of accommodations that a student with diabetes may qualify for, depending on that student's unique situation, which should be discussed with a health-care provider and the disability services coordinator at the school. The student may receive priority registration to make sure that he or she has the opportunity to register for classes that fit best with diabetes management. Similarly, the student may also receive assistance with attendance policies. The accommodations may include permission to bring food or drinks into a classroom and permission to leave the classroom to treat out-of-range blood sugar values in situations when these might not otherwise be permitted. The student may also receive assistance dealing with dining services to obtain nutritional information. Students may also elect to receive alternate testing opportunities for times when their blood glucose values are significantly out of range.

Along with proper accommodations, one of the most important things that parents can do is help students build the support network that will assist them in becoming successful adults with diabetes. (This book provides some program ideas in the resources section.) All young adults with and without diabetes are making decisions throughout college about their health and their behavior and the types of activities that influence their health. With proper encouragement and support, college can provide an opportunity for students to develop healthy diabetes management habits and decision-making processes.

Sara Nicastro has a Masters of Education in College Student Affairs and has worked in the field of higher education for more than 10 years. After a series of misdiagnoses, she was diagnosed with type 1 diabetes in 2003 in the midst her college experience. She is a passionate diabetes advocate and writes about her experiences living as an adult with diabetes on her web site at MomentsofWonderful.com.

Planning ahead and knowing how to handle it will help smooth the way.

The first thing you need to accept is this: it is up to your child to decide where he or she is going to school. While your input is certainly welcome, do not suggest that teens need to stay close to home because of their diabetes. Teens should choose a college based on their interests and desires (and what can be afforded!), not based on their diabetes. Remember, with e-mail and Internet, it's perfectly simple to keep an endocrinologist you see at home, even if your child is far away in college.

You'll want to discuss whether your child wants to register at the office of disabilities at college or not. College is not like grade school and high school: your child won't be filing a detailed plan on when he or she can start or stop testing because of highs or lows. New students won't be demanding a buddy to walk with them to the health office. In fact, whether or not children register or tell professors about their diabetes should be left totally up to them.

Sometimes registering is a good idea. If your child should end up with a long diabetes-related illness (say, one that requires hospitalization), that documentation could help in setting up make-up work instead of having to get a frustrating (and expensive) withdraw pass from a class. And one benefit that has little to do with diabetes: at many schools, students who are registered with a disabilities office get to register for classes earlier, giving them access to classes that may fill up quickly. Why not take the advantages when you can?

As for telling professors, it is up to your child. You might want the child to think about why a professor would need to know. In most cases, college students do not let professors know. By this age, they should be carrying their supplies and dealing with highs and lows on their own and with relative ease. And if they should end up sick, many want to just deal with it the same way anyone else who is sick has to. Some professors are understanding; some are not. It's all part of life.

As for telling a roommate, your teen does have an obligation to tell roommates right away that he or she has diabetes. They will be sharing a room; it's only fair the roommate knows right off that diabetes is onboard. But if your teen does not want to do the entire history of type 1, it's okay if they share something like "I wanted to let you know I have type 1 diabetes. I use an insulin pump and syringes and some other stuff. But I know what I am doing, and I never leave needles around or anything, so it's totally cool."

While some parents want to enlist the roommate as a substitute parent, training them in glucagon and low and high blood sugar detection, this is not fair. Let your child have a roommate experience without diabetes getting in the way—the same experience anyone else would have. It is okay to show the roommate where the glucagon is kept in the room and encourage them to call you (give the roommate your cell number) and 911 if need be. But beyond that, don't place all that on a roommate. In time if they become close, the roommate will want to learn. Let it evolve naturally.

As for whom to notify on the floor, it's not a bad idea for your teen to let the resident assistant know he or she has diabetes. If only in case of an emergency so the RA will know what is going on, this is a good idea.

The rest of it—the parties and the

> ### What about the Bad Roommate?
>
> This is a fear of all parents, not just parents of kids with diabetes. Your child does not have to be close friends with a roommate. They'll make friends in the hall and in classes. As long as they respect one another and live in peace, roommates work out fine. If a roommate is trouble, though, your child should talk to the resident assistant (RA). But they do not have to be best friends for things to go well.

A VISIT HOME FROM A COLLEGE TEEN'S PERSPECTIVE

Going to college with diabetes was something that was never questioned in my family, but I didn't realize how big of a change it would really be. I was on my own, and there was no one there to nag me except for those occasional calls (and Facebook messages, and tweets, and texts) from my mom where she'd ask me how everything was going. For the most part I transitioned well and got used to dealing with my daily diabetes care on my own.

I did miss my parents, my sister, and mostly my cat, but I did not miss my mother's diabetes oversight. By the time Thanksgiving came around, I couldn't wait to go home and visit. I eagerly waited for the day I'd fly home. I thought about my cat being curled up on my bed. I imagined laughing with my family.

What I didn't think about was the nagging.

When I was home my mom could see what was going on with my diabetes. When she sees what is going on she can't help but nag. It's human nature for a mother of a child with diabetes.

When the nagging began, I was not a happy camper. I was irritated with my mom asking "Did you bolus for that?" or "When was the last time you checked?" She and I have always had a great relationship, but the nagging irritated me more than anything. After a few days of rolling my eyes and ignoring her, we made a deal. The nagging would stop, and I would come to her and discuss my diabetes when I *wanted to*.

This compromise had to happen for a lot of reasons:

1. I was ready to be responsible, and I was old enough to be responsible. With that comes knowing when to ask for input and advice, and my mom had to understand that and trust that I would.
2. I was at school far away. I didn't see my mom as much, and I hated wasting time being upset or arguing. It would be better for us in every way if we could move past this.

Of course this not only meant my mom had to stop nagging, but it meant I had to work at not giving her reasons to nag. We both vowed to do those things.

Compromise is a big part of growing up, and Mom and I have always been about making it work for us. I realized from being away that when she couldn't nag me, she was happier and I was doing a better job of taking care of myself.

Now that I'm away and maturing, my diabetes care is better than it ever has been before. Every now and then, my mom will nag by accident, but as I said before, it is only her human nature, and it's a sign of being a good mom.

Now, when I come home, I still think about my cat curling up on my bed. I still look forward to laughing at all our funny family jokes, but I don't worry so much about the nagging.

It seems we've all grown up in our diabetes life from this college experience.

Lauren Stanford

checking and managing of diabetes and the balancing of classes and fun and sports and more—are all part of the process of growing up that you must, at this point, let your child experience and learn from. Mistakes will be made. Lessons will be learned. And hopefully, from all that will emerge a wonderful adult ready to take on the world.

Why Teens Should Have Hope

Someone told them years ago they'd see a cure in five years. Someone else promised that by the time they went to college, diabetes would be history. You are reading this, so that's not the case (and if it is, burn this book and celebrate!).

But teens have every reason to have hope in this life with diabetes.

First and foremost, they are most likely going to live long, healthy, full, and happy lives. The life expectancy for people with T1D is nearly the same as a person without it now. Sure, it's not as easy to live with diabetes as without, but live they will.

Second, better tools are on their way. Smarter pumps. Better insulin. CGMs that eventually remove the need to prick a finger. Teens can simply research a little and find that all of this is getting closer and closer to reality.

And if your teen is moving closer to adult years, they've passed through what may very well be the roughest time of all. Hormones, mood swings, fighting with parents, burnout, and even some scary times have passed. From all of it, they—and you—have grown, learned, and adapted.

They're ready to fly; with diabetes onboard, they're ready to fly.

Resources

Blogs

www.sixuntilme.com
Written by an adult with T1D who was diagnosed at age six, this site discusses daily living with diabetes in a down-to-earth way.

http://diabetesaliciousness.blogspot.com
Written by an adult with T1D, this site uses humor to share daily living with diabetes.

www.despitediabetes.com
This book's author's blog. Discussions on raising a child and young adult with T1D.

www.textingmypancreas.com
Information, advice, and insight from a woman who has grown up with T1D.

www.ourdiabeticlife.com
Wisdom and insight from a mom raising three boys with T1D (and one more without).

www.ninjabeetic.com
Life with diabetes from a man who is a father, worker, advocate, and person diagnosed as a teen.

www.scottsdiabetes.com
Insight from a man with T1D, honest input on eating issues, struggles, and successes.

www.diabetesmine.com
Written by a group of bloggers, this blog has become a go-to place for innovation information, advocacy, and tips on daily living with T1D.

Web Sites

www.childrenwithdiabetes.com
Perhaps the largest and most respected online diabetes community. Parents and teens alike can find information, guidance, and real-time support.

www.diabetesresearch.org
Located in Miami, Florida, the DRI has a research center focusing on the biological aspects of a cure, such as replacement therapy.

www.myglu.org
A combination of support system, information site, and data-gathering group (for research information), this site is a good go-to spot for lots of information and even some fun. Teens must have parental permission to access.

www.typeonenation.org
JDRF's online community, where you can find (or create) groups for all kinds of support and discussion.

Books

Transitions in Care: Meeting the Challenges of Type 1 Diabetes in Young Adults
(Howard Wolpert, MD; Barbara Anderson, PhD; Jill Weissberg-Benchell, PhD). *Transitions in Care* serves as a coaching manual for health-care providers and parents, and as a guide to self-care and independence for young adults with diabetes. It demystifies a complicated period in a life with type 1 diabetes and makes the passage to adulthood easier for everyone involved.

Emotional Eating with Diabetes
(Ginger Viera). This part book, part workbook guides you through eating challenges, from the mind of a woman who grew up with diabetes. Sidebars from folks who have been there add to the information.

Diabetes Burnout: What To Do When You Can't Take It Anymore
(William Polonsky, PhD). While this book was written back in 1999, it remains a go-to for insight and information on dealing with diabetes burnout.

The Discovery of Insulin
(Michael Bliss). A must-read that details the history and discovery of insulin and its use.

Think Like a Pancreas: A Practical Guide to Managing Diabetes with Insulin
(Gary Scheiner). Tips and details on managing insulin in the real world. Reads like your own CDE in a pocket.

Pumping Insulin: Everything You Need for Success with an Insulin Pump
(John Walsh): Called the "bible of pumping" by many, a good resource for all that is insulin pumping.

Programs

The Barton Center for Diabetes Education *www.bartoncenter.org* A leader in diabetes camping and educational programs.

Friends for Life: Annual conference held in Orlando each July by *www.childrenwithdiabetes.com*. Programs for parents, teens, siblings, and more. Other programs offered throughout the year as well, such as technology programs and overseas programs.

JDRF Advocacy Program *advocacy.jdrf.org* An easy way to get involved with programs and issues in Washington, D.C.

Riding on Insulin *ridingoninsulin.org* Camps held around the world annually for kids with diabetes who want to snowboard or ski. Run by world-class snowboarder and person with T1D Sean Busby.

Insulindependence *insulindepedence.org* National program for kids with diabetes who want to be active and adventurous. Events and leadership programs available.

Index

Employers, sharing diagnosis with, 40–41
Erectile dysfunction (ED), fear of, 23–24, 144
Estrogen, 17, 21
Exercise, 22, 23, 29, 93–94

F

Faking data, 56
Family dynamics
    diabetes diagnosis causing shift in, 81–82
    of extended family, 87, 89–90
    parents as role models, 92–94
    sibling factor in, 82–87
    with single parents, 90–92
Fear, 23–24, 83–84
Flexibility, promoting of, 38, 42, 87
Food and social life, 137–140
Freedom
    attitudes that mean trouble, 173
    free will and daily diabetes dares, 170–173
    meaning of to teens, 169–170
    teen and parental views of, 163–169
Friends
    "Diabetes World Friends," 109–110
    enlisting as helpers and supporters, 104–105, 135, 161, 243
    and long-diagnosed teens, 102–103
    making a difference, 106–107, 223
    and newly diagnosed teens, 100–102
    nonsocial or shy teens and, 106
    sharing diagnosis with, 36–37, 140
    temptation for parents "to use," 109
    who annoy, 107–109
"Friends for Life," 110
Friends for Life Conference, 229–230

G

George Mason University, 227
Girls
    growth spurts in, 26–27

menstrual cycles and glucose levels, 18–21, 25
    risk of pregnancy in, 141
    signs and average age of puberty, 17–18
    weight gain in, 21
Glucagon, 126, 161
Glucose (fast-acting), 150, 156
Glucostix, 150
Goal setting, 183–184
Gratitude, 60
Growth spurts, 26–27
Guidance counselors, 122
Guilt, 83, 89

H

Helping Students with Diabetes Succeed at College, 240–241
Hormones, 18, 22–23, 26

I

Independence
    See also Transitioning to self-care
    as developmental stage, 169–170
    with endo appointments, 209–211
    moving toward, 46, 51, 75, 113–114, 127
    never too early to get ready, 236–239
    responsibilities involved, 120, 126–127
    safely promoting, 172–173
    on school trips, 135
Insulin
    alcohol's impact on, 159, 160
    basal, 20, 65, 66, 67
    choices of, 63–64
    combinations of, 38
    contraception and, 144
    exercise aiding body's use of, 22
    hormones working against, 18, 21, 26
    injection sites, 31–32, 66
    long acting, 20, 26, 66

Acknowledgments

Writing a book is like having a baby. For months, it's all you think about, and everyone you even remotely know (sorry about my blabbering, cashiers at Skippy's Market) gets swept along, like it or not. With that, I have so many folks to thank for this book's completion and hopefully success. Such as: Katie and Steve Clark and family: anything I even pretend to know about life with diabetes I probably learned from you. D-Moms such as Meri, Katie Black, Ellen Ullman, Renee Bernett, Paula Fairchild, Michelle Crouse, Tanya Moder, the hilarious Michelle Weisenberg and so many more I could not list them all here, who guided me, made me laugh, and told me when I might have been wrong. Writer friends like Paula Ford–Martin, Lynn Prowitt, Allen St. John, Maggie Meade, and more who understand how cruel deadlines can be and why a girl truly needs a system of fake deadlines to survive. The person who invented Cool Lime Refreshers at Starbucks: I owe you big time, since this is my new fuel. Young adult friends with T1D such as Anna Floreen, Caroline McEnery, Kerri Sparling, Kelly Kunik, Krista Middleton and more, who not only have helped me understand all this, but have become a true resource to Lauren in her life as a young adult with T1D. Medical folks who have had our backs along the way, such as Dr. Dude, aka Dr. Jake Kushner, now of Texas Children's, Susan Crowell, and "Dr. Wonderful" himself, Dr. Howard Wolpert of Joslin. When I hear folks say they have a hard time getting in touch with their medical team or bonding with them, I scratch my head. You all have helped us become the educated, confident family we are and we will never forget that. (And I am sure you will recognize your advice over the years here in this book). The folks at CWD, particularly Jeffrey Hitchcock and Laura Billetdeaux, who helped me keep my voice when I thought I might be losing it, and who work endlessly for the good of so many. My good friends who knew when I needed a break and dragged me out for fun: The Bryants and the Hartnetts to name two of many. A special thank you to Anne D'Angelo for being such a good friend and listener even before she joined me in this D-Mom life. Brave parents, who have weathered the unimaginable and still spend every day helping others, such as Michelle Alswager and Duke Roos. You guys are true heroes to me, and I can only hope to be a tenth of the person each of you are. Folks in the diabetes professional world and/or non-profit world whom Lauren looks up to as a role model, such as Heidi Daniels, Laura Whitton, and the DCGR crew: I thank you for inspiring my former teen to make a difference in this world. And to my many, many friends in life from outside the diabetes world who are patient with me when I need to vent about all this, who take the time to learn and care and who donate every time I do something crazy like ride 100 miles across a desert in search of a cure. I have been truly blessed. Of course, there's Louie the Supercat. You kept my feet warm, listened patiently when I needed to read something aloud, and perched on the chair in my office just right. Thanks for being a furry, fun copilot. Last but so much on my mind and in my heart: My dear Caitlin. How I miss you every day. Every word of this book was written wishing I still had your humor, wisdom, and guidance to help me along. You are forever missed.

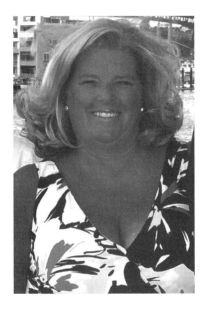

Moira McCarthy

Moira McCarthy is an acclaimed writer, author, and public speaker who has shared her story—and lessons—on raising a child with type 1 diabetes in the media, through books, and on her popular blog, *www.despitediabetes.com*. With over 15 years of experience raising a child with diabetes, McCarthy offers a frank, empowering perspective from a mother who has successfully weathered the teenage years and made it to the other side with a healthy, outstanding young adult.

McCarthy has appeared on *CNN Live*, *Good Morning America*, *Fox News*, and in *The New York Times*. She was recently recognized as the JDRF International Volunteer of the Year. Her six books include the top-selling *Everything Parents Guide to Juvenile Diabetes*.